Fixed Prosthodontics in Dental Practice

Quintessentials of Dental Practice – 22
Prosthodontics - 4

Fixed Prosthodontics in Dental Practice

By
Michael O'Sullivan

Editor-in-Chief: Nairn H F Wilson
Editor Prosthodontics: P Finbarr Allen

Quintessence Publishing Co. Ltd.
London, Berlin, Chicago, Paris, Milan, Barcelona, Istanbul,
São Paulo, Tokyo, New Delhi, Moscow, Prague, Warsaw

British Library Cataloguing-in Publication Data

O'Sullivan, Michael
  Fixed prosthodontics in dental practice. - (Quintessentials of dental practice ; 22.
  Prosthodontics ; 4)
  1. Prosthodontics
  I. Title II. Wilson, Nairn H. F. III. Allen, P. Finbarr
  617.6´9

ISBN 1850970955

ISBN 1-85097-095-5

Foreword

Good quality, aesthetically pleasing fixed prosthodontics that fulfil patient expectations are a potent, professionally rewarding practice builder. Achieving consistently high standards in fixed prosthodontics is, however, a substantial challenge, even for the experienced practitioner. This challenge may be best managed by having a good understanding of the evolving principles of modern fixed prosthodontics, underpinned by up-to-date knowledge of contemporary techniques and relevant materials.

Fixed Prosthodontics in Dental Practice, Volume 22 of the timely *Quintessentials of Dental Practice* series, meets this need. It is not intended to be a comprehensive tome; it is a succinct, authoritative overview of the key elements of fixed prosthodontics, with a focus on achieving good clinical outcomes. This book, in common with all the other volumes of the *Quintessentials* series, makes easy reading over an evening or two and has been prepared in a style to encourage readers to rethink their current approach - in this case, to fixed prosthodontics. From patient assessment through to the evaluation of completed restorations, this carefully crafted, attractively illustrated, multi-author text provides sound, evidence-based guidance, tempered by a wealth of experience shared by experts in the field.

This book provides new insight for students of all ages - yet another excellent addition to the very popular and rapidly expanding *Quintessentials of Dental Practice* series.

Nairn Wilson
Editor-in-Chief

Preface

The practice of fixed prosthodontics has undergone many changes in recent times, with significant developments in dental materials and principles of adhesion. However, tooth preparation is still guided by the need to preserve tooth tissue, generate space for restorative material and reshape the tooth to a cylindrical form with a defined finish line. This book carries these principles as a common theme and delineates how it influences the steps of prosthesis construction.

It is intended to act as a guide that supplements existing prosthodontic knowledge and focuses on areas that are traditionally covered in less detail, such as assessment, shade-taking, assessment of completed restorations and decision-making for restoration of non-vital teeth.

It is hoped that having read this book the reader will have an increased understanding of:
- The importance of patient assessment, with emphasis on assessment of abutments, edentulous spaces and occlusal forces.
- Principles of preparation and how restorative space will have a significant impact on the success of both conventional and adhesive prostheses.
- How periodontal factors and operating field control can enhance prosthetic outcomes.
- The importance and multiple functions of provisional prostheses.
- How correct simulation of maxillo-mandibular relations can improve the final prosthesis and reduce clinical time spent adjusting restorations.
- The challenges of colour-matching ceramics and how to improve colour communication with the dental technician.
- How to evaluate a completed prosthesis in a step-wise fashion.
- How to choose a luting agent.
- Decision-making in restoring endodontically treated teeth.

Michael O'Sullivan

Acknowledgements

I would like to thank my colleagues at the Dublin Dental Hospital for their support in the preparation of this book. In particular I would like to thank Dr. Finbarr Allen for his editorial assistance and Professor Liam McDevitt, Dr. Frank Quinn and Professor Brian O'Connell for their ideas and encouragement. I would like to thank all the contributors to the individual chapters who toiled without complaint. The authors reflect a wide spectrum of prosthodontic backgrounds, which is helpful in establishing a consensus of opinion.

Finally I would like to thank Noreen, Fionn and Joe for their collective proof-reading and patience over the time it has taken to complete this book.

Contributors

Dr. Michael O'Sullivan	Senior Lecturer /Consultant, Department of Restorative Dentistry & Periodontology, Dublin Dental School & Hospital, Dublin, Ireland
Edward G. Owens	Private practitioner, practice limited to prosthodontics, Dublin 6
Dr. Paul Quinlan	Lecturer, Department of Restorative Dentistry & Periodontology, Dublin Dental School & Hospital, Dublin, Ireland and Private practitioner, practice limited to prosthodontics, Dublin 2
Dr. R. Gerard Cleary	Lecturer, Department of Restorative Dentistry & Periodontology, Dublin Dental School & Hospital, Dublin, Ireland and Private practitioner, practice limited to prosthodontics, Dublin 4
Dr. Kevin O'Boyle	Private practitioner, practice limited to prosthodontics, Dublin 4
Prof William E. McDevitt	Professor /Consultant, Department of Restorative Dentistry & Periodontology, Dublin Dental School & Hospital, Dublin, Ireland
Dr. John Fearon	Postgraduate, Department of Restorative Dentistry & Periodontology, Dublin Dental School & Hospital, Dublin, Ireland
Dr. Frank Quinn	Senior Lecturer /Consultant, Department of Restorative Dentistry & Periodontology, Dublin Dental School & Hospital, Dublin, Ireland
Prof. Brian O'Connell	Professor /Consultant, Department of Restorative Dentistry & Periodontology, Dublin Dental School & Hospital, Dublin, Ireland

Contents

Chapter 1
Patient Assessment and Presentation of Treatment Options

Aim

The aim of this chapter is to outline the process from initial patient contact to arrival at a treatment plan. An algorithm is suggested to assist methodical data collection and diagnosis.

Outcome

After reading this chapter, the clinician should be able to provide a framework within which to accumulate and interpret clinical findings in order to formulate a relevant treatment plan for individual patients.

Introduction

During the first consultation, both the patient's presenting complaint and its history should be recorded in the patient's own words and be as detailed as possible. The record should act as a focus during examination, and the final treatment option must fully address this complaint. A record must be made of any previous treatment for the same complaint to assist in the analysis of success or failure. A complete patient record consists of three phases:
- patient history
- dental examination
- special tests.

Patient History

A complete patient history should include:
- *Dental history* – a record of past attendance, treatments and associated complications following treatment. It should address any history of trauma and reasons for extraction of teeth. The former is significant as teeth may, as a consequence, be compromised, and the prognosis for treatment involving these teeth can be less favourable. Loss of teeth may be an indicator of caries or periodontal disease susceptibilities and suggest difficulties with replacement of missing teeth from ongoing caries or soft tissue recession and attachment loss.

- *Medical history* – this can be recorded using a variety of methods, but before treatment the following questions must be addressed:
  - Will any element of the patient's medical history affect dental treatment?
  - Will any element of the patient's dental treatment affect his or her medical status?
  - Is the patient taking any medication that will affect dental treatment?
  - Will dental treatments affect the patient's current medication regimen (including prescription medication)?
- *Social history* - provides a background to the patient and identifies habits (for example, smoking and alcohol consumption) or pastimes (for instance, contact sports or hobbies involving hyperbaric conditions) that may influence treatment options.

Dental Examination

A dental examination should address:
- *Disease* - the first step in preparation for prosthodontic treatment is to identify and eliminate disease in order to establish health. Disease should encompass both past experience and current status.
- *Periodontal health* - a complete periodontal examination identifies the current status of the supporting tissues. Active disease must be addressed prior to prosthodontic treatment. The periodontal examination should also highlight areas that influence treatment outcome, such as teeth with furcation involvement or poor prognosis. The effects of previous periodontal disease should be taken into consideration - in particular, attachment loss and resulting recession, tooth mobility, irregular gingival margin heights and the absence of attached gingivae in any area (see Chapter 3). Effectiveness of home dental care should also be assessed and modified, if necessary, prior to definitive treatment planning (Fig 1-1).
- *Caries assessment* - this should identify existing lesions and restorations present. The number and extent of restorations indicates past caries experience, and location may suggest rampant caries if the mandibular incisors or mandibular lingual surfaces are restored. Based on this exam, a preventative regimen can be targeted to the individual patient's needs.
- *Pulpal health* – the pulpal health of individual teeth should be assessed if they are heavily restored or have been traumatised. Tests should include cold/hot/electric pulp testing, in addition to percussion and radiographs. Findings from retrospective studies have determined that many prosthodontic failures occurred as a result of having to complete endodontic treatment after placement of the definitive prosthesis, so careful preoperative

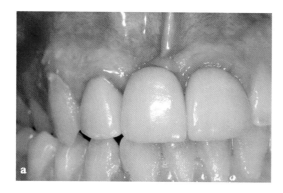

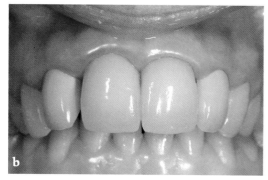

Fig 1-1 Periodontal tissue breakdown, as a result of (a) poor local hygiene or (b) iatrogenic causes.

assessment is necessary. If teeth are endodontically treated, the following questions should be addressed:
- Is the tooth restorable?
- Are there signs or symptoms of periapical inflammation?
- Is there associated pain?
- Radiographically is there an intact lamina dura and is there apical bone loss?
- If pathology is identified, is it resolving, static or worsening (Fig 1-2)?
- Is the canal obturation homogenous, well condensed and extending throughout the length of the canal?

If concerns exist about the status of an existing endodontic treatment then re-treatment, or extraction, should be considered.
• *Mucosal health* – the oral mucosa must be healthy before restorative treatment. Loss of mucosal continuity or discomfort must be controlled prior to definitive treatment planning. Such conditions include areas of ulcera-

3

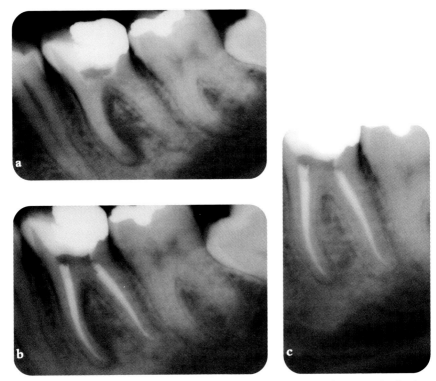

Fig 1-2 Endodontic treatments must demonstrate resolution of periapical infection prior to restoration of teeth. (a) Pre-op radiograph of tooth 36. (b) Immediate post-op radiograph. (c) Three month post-op recall radiograph, demonstrating resolution of the apical pathology.

tion or erosion, allergies and altered sensation such as 'burning mouth syndrome'. Consultation with an oral physician may be required to treat the condition prior to restorative care. If the mucosal condition is not controlled it will cause discomfort during treatment and may hinder oral hygiene procedures, making treatment and its maintenance more difficult.

• *Craniomandibular articulation (CMA) health* – a screening examination for joint derangement and muscle dysfunction must be completed to determine the need for more extensive investigation. The proposed screening exam acts as a good patient record and also brings any functional deficits to attention at an early stage (Table 1-1).

Table 1-1 **Craniomandibular articulation health exam**

1. Anterior tooth relationships: Class I, II, III (vertical and horizontal overlap).
2. Number of functional units in maximum intercusping position (MIP).
3. History of:
  (i) CMA noise, locking, pain
  (ii) muscle fatigue /discomfort
  (iii) difficulty in opening mouth, chewing, talking.
4. Tooth measurements.

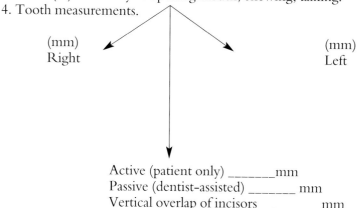

  (mm)   (mm)
  Right   Left

    Active (patient only) _____mm
    Passive (dentist-assisted) _____ mm
    Vertical overlap of incisors _____ mm
    Horizontal overlap of incisors _____ mm

5. Co-ordination of voluntary movements:
  depression: good, poor
  left lateral: good, poor
  right lateral: good, poor.

The CMA screening exam should address the following questions:
- Does a satisfactory end-stop exist in the MIP? Are there sufficient numbers and distribution of functional units?
- Are the overlap relationships/dynamic occlusions/anterior guidance satisfactory? Can they be improved?
- Is the patient excessively clenching or grinding the teeth? Does this pose a difficulty for the proposed treatment plan?
- Is there evidence of tooth mobility or fremitus? Is there evidence of damage in the dentition as a result of parafunction?
- Are teeth/CMA being overloaded?
- Is there evidence of intracapsular discomfort/pain during function or during the testing mandibular movements and/or manipulations?

- Is the range of mandibular depression and CMA comfort adequate for restorative procedures to be completed on posterior teeth over long treatment sessions?
- Is further functional assessment of the CMA status required? If the answer is yes, a more detailed examination/referral to a specialist practitioner is indicated.

Special Tests

Mechanics

Mechanics can be subdivided into micro- and macromechanics. These are best evaluated in conjunction with mounted study casts of the patient.

Micromechanics

Micromechanics are concerned with individual teeth and, in particular, proposed abutments. The strength of any individual crown is primarily determined by the amount of dentine remaining coronal to the finish line. The main features of the preparation include height, width and irregularity and are summarised in Table 1-2.

Table 1-2 **The micromechanical factors involved in determining the suitability of a tooth to receive a fixed restoration**

Prognosis	Excellent		Unfavourable
Amount of dentine	Intact	Restorations	Post/core
Preparation height	Tall		<3 mm
Preparation width	Narrow		Wide
Preparation irregularity	Irregular		Regular
Root shape	Splayed		Conical
Root length	Long		Short
Attachment level	No attachment loss		Less than 1:1

- *Height* - the greater the distance from the finish line of the preparation to the occlusal surface/incisal edge, the more difficult it is to dislodge an extracoronal restoration (Fig 1-3). Tipping forces on short preparations will result in poorly tolerated shear stress being placed on the luting agent, while on tall preparations it will result in more favourable compressive loading of the luting agent. Methods of improving preparation height include periodontal crown-lengthening, orthodontic extrusion or moving the finish line apically without encroaching on the biological width.

- *Width* - a narrow preparation has a smaller rotational path of dislodgement than a wider one. The inclusion of auxiliary retention should be borne in mind at the preparation stage. This includes axial slots, grooves and boxes that serve to decrease the radius of the rotational path of dislodgement (width/height relationship).

- *Irregularity* - a symmetrical smooth preparation will resist rotation less than an irregular preparation.

- *Root structure* - longer splayed roots are better able to resist occlusal forces and demonstrate reduced mobility in the event of attachment loss when compared to conical short roots (Fig 1-4). This becomes more critical when the tooth is to be used as an abutment.

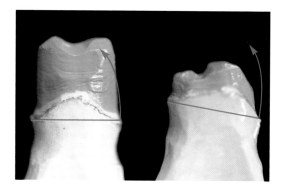

Fig 1-3 Effect of preparation height on loading of luting agents. Tipping forces on short preparations will result in poorly tolerated shear stress being placed on the luting agent, while on tall preparations will result in more favourable compressive loading of the luting agent.

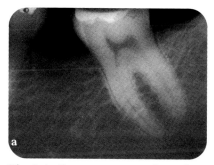 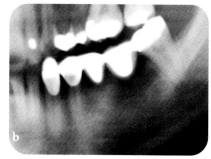

Fig 1-4 Root structure and attachment level. (a) Longer splayed roots without attachment loss provide preferable support for fixed restorations. (b) Short, conical roots and teeth that have lost attachment may reduce the ability of the tooth to resist occlusal forces, particularly when used as abutment for fixed partial dentures.

- *Attachment level* – the optimal tooth for prosthodontic purposes is one without attachment loss. Any loss is a compromise, in particular if there is a differential in mobility between abutments for a fixed partial denture. Attachment loss may also result in soft tissue loss. It is important to consider this, both aesthetically and from the preparation finish-line perspective, which may be on cementum – thought to be less favourable than preparations ending on enamel. In addition, as the finish line moves apically from the cemento-enamel junction the diameter of the tooth decreases. This may lead to increased risk of pulpal encroachment and the inability to reduce the required tooth tissue for restoration. Surgical crown lengthening may, however, be indicated if insufficient preparation height exists (see Chapter 3).

Macromechanics
This primarily involves occlusion but also includes edentulous spans in the case of fixed partial dentures. The probable functional and parafunctional occlusal load should be assessed both statically and dynamically. The edentulous span should be assessed under the following headings:

- *Parallelism of abutments* – if the proposed abutments diverge or are rotated, then additional tooth reduction will be required to ensure a common path of insertion. This additional tooth loss may damage the pulp. To manage divergence or convergence, consider a fixed-movable design, elective devitalisation of an abutment or orthodontic alignment.
- *Length of span* – beam law dictates that if the span of a beam is doubled then its flexibility increases eight times. Increasing metal bulk in the restoration or using an alloy with superior mechanical properties (for example, increased proportional limit and modulus of elasticity) will reduce flexure. To facilitate an appropriate pontic form, the dimensions of the edentulous span should be appropriate for the tooth/teeth being replaced. This is best assessed using a diagnostic wax-up. Orthodontic tooth movement may be indicated to improve proportions.
- *Occlusal factors* – in addition to requiring mesiodistal space, the pontic requires adequate vertical space (Figs 1-5 and 1-6). The pontic will have to compensate for any discrepancy in the opposing occlusal plane. It may result in a poor maximum intercusping relationship or compromised aesthetics. Furthermore, an overerupted tooth increases the risk of deflective contacts in lateral and protrusive movements. These deflective contacts generate horizontal shear stresses that are poorly tolerated by luting agents.

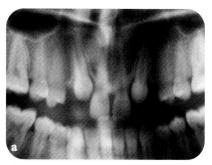
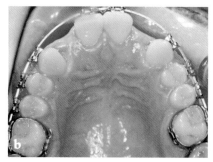

Fig 1-5 Inadequate mesio-distal width for a pontic site. (a) Insufficient mesio-distal space exists for prosthetic replacement of congenitally missing maxillary lateral incisors. (b) Creation of sufficient space is best achieved through orthodontic treatment.

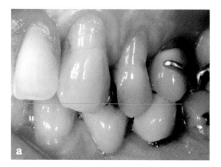
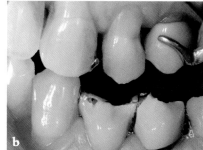

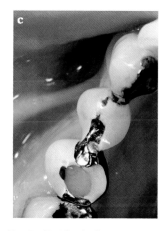

Fig 1-6 Inadequate vertical space for a pontic site. (a–b) As a result of over-eruption of teeth 23 and 24 the pontic on the FPD from 35 to 33 has to compensate for the discrepancy in the occlusal plane (red line). (c) This results in an unaesthetic pontic and increases the risk of occlusal interferences.

Aesthetic Considerations

Aesthetics are examined both in the face and smile. Individual observations in each area should be noted to complete a problem list. When assessing aesthetic appearance in the face, the following questions should be addressed:

9

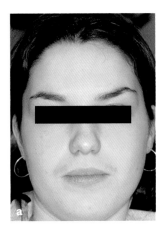 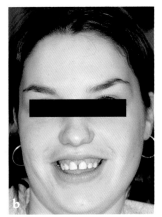

Fig 1-7 Level of lip at repose and smiling. A very mobile upper lip that demonstrates marked movement from (a) repose to (b) full smile poses more of an aesthetic challenge for restoration of anterior teeth.

- Is the lower third face height equal to the middle third face height (facial proportion)? Is there a skeletal problem?
- Is the distance from the lips to the chin twice that to the base of the nose? Is there lower face height loss?
- Is the upper lip of normal length (norm: males = 22-24 mm, females = 20-22 mm)? If the lips are short more tooth will be visible, which may complicate the aesthetic result.

When assessing aesthetic appearance in the teeth and smile of the patient, the following questions need addressing:
- What is the patient's perception?
- Is the patient happy with his or her dental appearance?
- Are the patient's expectations achievable?
- Is a multidisciplinary approach required?
- Is the maxillary midline correct relative to the centre line of the face or centre of the philtrum of the upper lip? Significant deviations may not be correctable by dental restorations alone.
- What teeth are visible in repose and full smile (Fig 1-7)? Is this appropriate for the age of the patient? (In repose a young female should show 3-4 mm and a male 1-2 mm of the maxillary anterior teeth).
- How far distally can be seen in repose and full smile, and is it symmetrical?
- There are four aesthetic indicators notable in relation to the dentition:
  - *Colour* - note teeth both individually and collectively.
  - *Dimension* - are the teeth of normal shape/height/width? Compare values with standard values and also check for symmetry of tooth form (Figs 1-8 and 1-9). If the teeth are short, is it as a result of tooth wear, para-

Fig 1-8 Position and dimension of teeth. Problems with the restoration on tooth 11 include its increased mesio-distal width, lack of symmetry, uneven gingival margins and poor colour match. Orthodontic alignment of the teeth and provision of a new restoration are indicated.

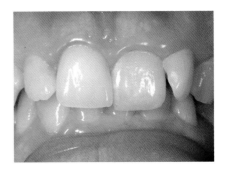

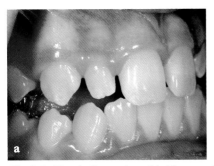
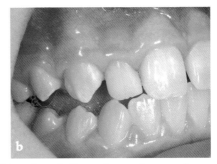

Fig 1-9 Tooth dimension. (a) Abnormalities of tooth dimension such as peg laterals need to assessed and restoration planned. (b) The width of the maxillary lateral incisor in this 12-year-old patient was increased from 4 to 6mm to facilitate orthodontic alignment and maintain space for later definitive restoration of the tooth. Note that the tooth alignment was not altered to facilitate uprighting of the tooth.

function or altered passive eruption? If the latter is suspected, probe for the amelocemental junction. If it cannot be located aesthetic crown-lengthening should be considered prior to restoration.

- *Position* - this relates to lip function and smile. Are the teeth in their correct orientation mesiodistally, buccolingually and in relation to the upper lip? Is tooth movement required?

- *Proportion* - Gillen and co-workers described proportions found in unworn maxillary dentitions. Central incisors and canines were of equal length, being 20% longer than the lateral incisor. The central incisor was wider than the lateral (25%) and canine (10%), and the length to width ratio of the lateral incisors and canines was 1.2:1, whereas the central incisor was 1.1:1.

Risk Analysis

Risk analysis considers potential problems relative to their probability and provision for failure. Potential problems are classified into biological, mechanical, aesthetic and patient factors. These category areas should be examined critically for potential difficulties during and after completion of treatment. Based on this analysis of risks and the highlighting of potential problems, many factors can be addressed through the use of alternative methods and materials. Common areas for consideration in each category are as follows:

- *Biological:*
  - Caries risk (based on past caries experience of patient and response to treatment).
  - Periodontal disease risk (based on prior experience of patient and response to treatment).
  - Endodontic risk (abutments becoming non-vital, post/core failure, endodontic failure, root fracture).
  - Occlusal risks (CMA effects).
  - Effects of parafunction (increased loading on restorations).
- *Mechanical:*
  - Cementation failure.
  - Restoration fracture.
  - Abutment fracture.
  - Effects of wear.
  - Risk of trauma (contact sports).
- *Aesthetic:*
  - Can the proposed result be obtained and maintained?
  - Are soft-tissue changes likely (for instance, recession)?
  - How will wear affect the restorations to be placed?
- *Patient factors:*
  - Expectations.
  - Dental awareness.
  - Achievability of goals.
  - Means.

Risk analysis highlights potential problems and helps reduce these risks through the use of alternative methods and materials.

Diagnostic Wax-Up

Completion of a diagnostic wax-up on mounted study casts prior to prosthodontic treatment (Fig. 1-10) has many advantages:

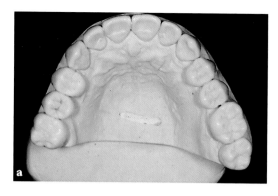

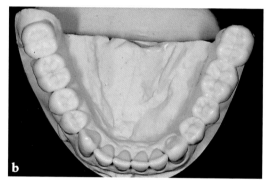

Fig 1-10 Diagnostic wax-up. (a) Maxillary aspect. (b) Mandibular aspect. A diagnostic wax-up provides a blueprint for any planned treatment and is essential where the shape and form of the teeth are being altered.

- It acts as a blueprint for the definitive prosthesis and provisional restorations.
- It may highlight three-dimensional (3D) problems involving occlusal relations. These can then be modified if necessary.
- It can be modified to provide additional information to the dental technician to assist in prosthesis construction.
- It can be used as a tooth preparation guide if axial or occlusal contours are to be altered in the definitive prosthesis.
- It can be shared with the patient prior to treatment, providing an indication of the anticipated outcome. In addition, it may be used to educate a patient in recognising the limitations of treatment.

Contingency Planning

This deals with planning for possible adverse outcomes at the treatment-planning stage. Key questions to be addressed are:
- In the event of failure of a component of treatment (identified by risk

assessment) are options available to facilitate later retreatment – for example, the inclusion of rest seats and guide planes in an extracoronal restoration adjacent to a proposed site for dental implants where the conditions for integration are not ideal?

- Can restorations be made to accommodate anticipated problems with tooth wear – for example, planning for wear of a natural maxillary canine prior to placement of cast premolar units to accommodate group function?
- Are there intermediate steps that can be included in patient treatment that allow the plan to be altered before definitive restoration? In the case of a long-span fixed partial denture, would placement of a laboratory-constructed provisional for a period of months indicate the long-term survival possibilities of the definitive restoration? If the provisional outcome is poor, then a fixed option may not be advisable.

The completion of risk analysis on proposed treatment options should permit an informed decision to be made as to the optimum course of action.

Conclusion

The provision of an optimal treatment plan for individual patients has many facets. In addition to the interpretation of clinical findings, any plan must assess the desires and expectations of the patient, limitations of restorations and the potential longevity and predictability of treatment. An algorithm is outlined to provide a logical sequence to patient assessment and presentation of treatment options.

Further Reading

Gillen RJ, Schwartz RS, Hilton TJ, Evans DB. An analysis of selected normative tooth proportions. Int J Prosthodont 1994;7:410-417.

Kokich VO Jr, Kiyak HA, Shapiro PA. Comparing the perception of dentists and lay people to altered dental esthetics. J Esthet Dent 1999;11:311-324.

Pameijer JHN. Periodontal and Occlusal Factors in Crown and Bridge Procedures. Holland: Dental Center for Postgraduate Courses, 1985:17-60.

Robbins JW. Esthetic considerations in diagnosis and treatment planning. In: Summitt JB, Robbins JW, Schwartz RS. Fundamentals of Operative Dentistry. 2nd Edn. Quintessence Publishing Co. Inc., 2001:56-70.

Rosenstiel SF, Ward DH, Rashid RG. Dentists' preferences of anterior tooth proportion – a web-based study. J Prosthodont 2000;9:123-136.

Chapter 2
Objectives of Tooth Preparation

Aim

Understanding the basic concepts and applying established principles of preparation procedures provides for more predictable outcomes in diverse clinical situations. This chapter reviews the key principles of tooth preparation.

Outcome

After reading this chapter, the clinician should be familiar with various concepts and principles of tooth preparation that have evolved through clinical practice and research. The reader will understand the importance of tooth preparation requiring conservation of as much sound tooth structure as possible, while providing adequate space for a predictable restoration.

Concepts and Principles

The fundamental aim of tooth preparation is to transform the tooth by a planned process to a uniformly reduced geometrical cylindrical form with a clearly defined finish line, permitting sufficient space for the mechanical and aesthetic properties of the planned restorative material. Successful tooth preparation will create a tooth shape that will allow for the optimal performance of the restoration complex, which includes the tooth preparation, luting material and the laboratory-fabricated extracoronal restoration.

Preparation Objectives

Tooth reduction for full coverage restorations must be consistent with individual tooth health, anatomy and dimension while meeting mechanically driven retention and resistance requirements for indirect restorations. Ensuring minimal damage to vital pulp tissue, adjacent teeth and soft tissues during the preparation procedure involves preoperative evaluation of the tooth and its immediate environment. Dimension and orientation vertically, mesiodistally and buccolingually, pulp size and gingival contours need to be considered prior to reduction procedures.

Analysis of preoperative study casts provides the necessary information on tooth dimension, angulation and alignment within the arch and an appreciation of gingival contour. Radiographs provide information on root form and pulp chamber shape and size.

Modifications are planned in the preparation in accordance with the ultimate role of the restoration. Requirements vary if the preparation is for an abutment for a removable or fixed partial denture as opposed to a single crown. Examples of modifications include rest seat preparation, guide planes, fixed movable joints and parallelism of abutments.

Objectives can be considered under the headings of biological, mechanical and aesthetic factors.

Biological Considerations
The biological significance of tooth reduction needs to be evaluated in terms of:
- Maintenance of pulp vitality and maximising potential for tissue conservation through anatomic reduction.
- Maintenance of the integrity of adjacent teeth and soft tissues.

Pulp Health and Tissue Conservation
Vital teeth are subject to pulpal insult during preparation. The following factors act in combination to affect pulpal health:
- *Temperature* - excessive heat generation can lead to pulpal injury and must be kept to a minimum.
- *Instrumentation* - appropriate bur selection and sequencing will increase the efficiency of the preparation procedure and reduce the risks of pulpal insult. Bulk reduction will require a diamond coarse-cut bur of adequate dimension while the final shape may be accomplished with finer-grit diamond burs.
- *Desiccation* - this can lead to severe pulpal irritation, therefore prepared teeth should be kept moist during the cutting procedures with adequate cooled water spray.
- *Age* - the thickness of the remaining dentine is inversely proportional to the pulpal response to tooth preparation. Minimal preparation of the tooth to create the optimal occlusal convergence angle between the walls of the preparation will reduce pulpal insult.
- *Non-uniform tooth reduction due to alignment problems* - this may lead to excessive tooth reduction and pulp exposure. This can be more significant where alignment discrepancies are to be corrected or if the tooth is to serve

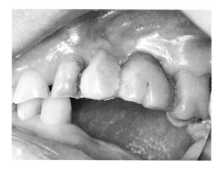

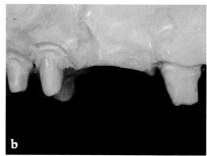

Fig 2-1 Alignment difficulties for fixed partial dentures. (a) Over-eruption and rotations on teeth such as 2.6 pose significant difficulties for tooth preparation. (b) Additional reduction may be required to correct angulation difficulties. (c) Definitive prosthesis on verification cast.

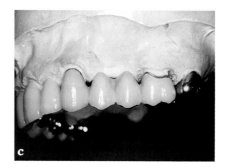

as a fixed partial denture abutment. Where a combination of vital and non-vital abutments exists, vital abutments should be prepared first, followed by preparations on non-vital teeth (Fig 2-1). This limits the excessive reduction and pulpal insult to vital teeth while satisfying alignment requirements.

Adequate occlusal reduction is required to allow sufficient space for developing a functional occlusal scheme in the final restoration. Reduction along anatomic planes provides for a more conservative approach.

More extensive preparations (for example, all-ceramic crowns) will require more circumferential and occlusal tooth reduction than preparations for metal ceramic restorations, due to material requirements.

Shoulder, shoulder with bevel and chamfer finishes have been studied and all three configurations were found to be unrelated to the fit of cemented crowns. All-ceramic restorations have definite chamfer/rounded shoulder finish-line requirements.

Adjacent Tissues

The pre- and perioperative management of the gingival tissues is essential for effective tooth preparation and impression-making. The finish line should be placed at a level consistent with gingival health and preservation of the biologic width (Fig 2-2). Ideally, the finish line should be at, or above, the gingival margin. Sometimes it is necessary to extend the finish line to eliminate caries or existing restorations. Aesthetic demands may also necessitate the subgingival placement of finish lines.

Tissues may need to be modified prior to preparation to meet this requirement and allow creation of a definite finish line.

Appropriate bur selection and attention to handpiece alignment is necessary to limit the risks of damaging adjacent tooth structure during tooth preparation procedures. This is especially significant where access is limited and use of a paediatric handpiece may provide more control in these situations.

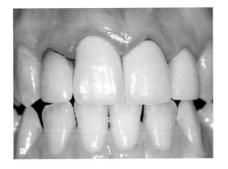

Fig 2-2 Biological width encroachment. (a) Unaesthetic anterior restorations with subgingival margins and resultant gingival inflammation. (b) Radiograph of the showing location of margins. (c) Close-up view of area between teeth 11 and 21. The finish lines of the preparation are within 1mm of the bone crest, and insufficient space exists between the roots of the teeth. A combination orthodontic/periodontal and restorative treatment is required for success of future restorations.

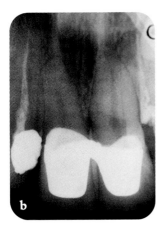

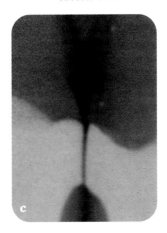

Mechanical Considerations

The objective of tooth preparation is to create adequate geometry, incorporating an optimal total convergence angle without undercuts. This provides a single path of placement and sufficient resistance and retention form within the body of the preparation to sustain the appropriate foundation for the restoration. Accuracy of fit in terms of crown adaptation to a geometrically favourable tooth preparation will limit the stress delivered to the cementing medium and contributes to maintaining the integrity of the cement lute.

Retention and Resistance Form

Retention form is the quality inherent in a crown to resist vertical forces of dislodgement. Retention is primarily a phenomenon of the geometrical form of the preparation. The features of a tooth preparation that enhance the stability and resist rotation from the seated position are the resistance form. These features limit the most damaging stresses delivered to cemented restorations in clinical situations, namely forces exerted in lateral and horizontal directions (Table 2-1).

Table 2-1 **Factors influencing the retention and resistance of a preparation**

Convergence angle	6-10 degrees ideally
	14-27 degrees is commonly found in practice
Axial preparation height	Minimum 3mm for anterior teeth
	Minimum 4mm for posterior teeth
	Increase through crown-lengthening surgery or orthodontic extrusion
Height to width ratio	>0.4 required as a guide
Circumferential irregularity	Achieved through anatomical reduction and preservation of line angles to avoid a rounded preparation
Surface roughness	Retention of a restoration may be enhanced by a rough surface; this must be offset against the difficulty in seating a restoration due to resistance to cement flow
Auxillary retentive features	Can significantly augment deficiencies in the retention and resistance require ments by improving resistance form

Mechanical Preparation Guidelines
The relationship between total convergence angle, axial wall height and circumferential morphology has been identified as the significant factor affecting retention and resistance properties of the tooth preparation.

Finish Line
A well-defined smooth and even finish line is necessary to provide marginal integrity and facilitate accurate fit of the crown restoration. The finish line must be located on sound tooth structure, not plastic restorations or unsupported enamel. Manual checking of the margin with a curette or ultrasonic instrumentation is necessary to ensure the finish-line requirements are met and unsupported enamel removed.

The configuration of the finish line for metal ceramic restorations has been found to be equally effective as a shoulder, shoulder bevel or chamfer. Choice of specific configuration of finish line is a matter of preference and related to aesthetic requirements and ease of formation (Fig 2-3). Ensuring adequate tooth tissue reduction to provide space for sufficient material bulk of ceramic or metal-ceramic veneering material and to prevent structural material weakness relating to a loss of rigidity is essential. Reduced space also compromises restoration thickness and can lead to aesthetic compromise and overcontouring of the final restoration.

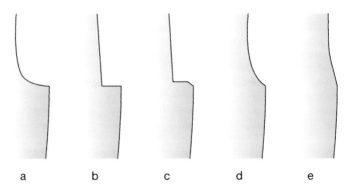

    a   b   c   d   e

Fig 2-3 Finish lines for cast restorations. (a) Deep chamfer (b) Shoulder (c) Shoulder-bevel (d) Chamfer (e) Feather edge.

Aesthetic Considerations

Aesthetic variables include colour, position, dimension and proportion. Considerations involve whether anomalies can be corrected in a predictable manner with the selected restoration or whether other adjunctive treatments need to be provided initially. The dimension of the prepared tooth core will need to be visualised to prevent over-contouring of the final restoration.

• Tooth reduction - facial axial reduction of 1.2-1.5mm for metal-ceramic and 1.0-1.2mm for all-ceramic crowns is recommended. Occlusal reductions of up to 2mm can be achieved without significant compromise to pulpal health. However, these are guidelines, and previous restorative history of the tooth can have a significant effect on pulpal conditions and the ability to provide adequate tooth reduction without compromising tooth vitality. Significant vertical reduction for aesthetic reasons can, of course, compromise the potential for developing retention and resistance form in the tooth preparation.

• Space for restorative material - reduced restoration thickness resulting from inadequate tooth reduction can lead to aesthetic compromise and overcontouring of the final restoration. Adequate reduction is required to provide space for sufficient material bulk of ceramic or metal-ceramic veneering material. Reduction should be biplanar (Fig 2-4).

• Marginal placement - aesthetic requirements and the condition of the tooth will determine the finish-line location. When subgingival finish lines are required they should not be extended to the epithelial attachment. The type of material used in the construction of the restoration will determine the configuration of the finish line. Preparation in aesthetically critical situations may require two or more treatment appointments to accomplish. Completed initial preparation and provisionalisation is followed by preparation finessing and impression-making at a subsequent treatment appointment. This will allow for more objective evaluation of the level of the finish line with respect to tissue response to the provisional restoration, prior to making a final impression.

• Gingival factors - the tooth dimension and gingival relationship must be conducive to an acceptable aesthetic result. Occlusocervical dimensions, tooth symmetry and gingival aesthetics are affected by gingival levels, thickness and contour in the cervical area. Non-vital teeth that have discoloured will place significant constraints on the ability to deliver aesthetic outcomes and affect the level of the finish line placement and depth of tooth reduction required (Fig 2-5). These factors are of much greater significance in high smile-line patients with knife-edge, thin gingival tissue and patients with gingival recession. In such patient groups the emergence profile requirements in the devel-

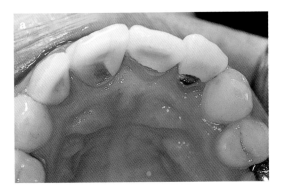

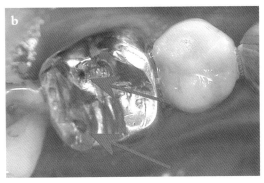

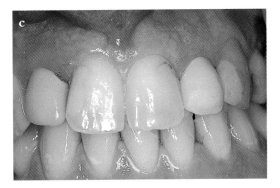

Fig 2-4 Insufficient tooth reduction commonly resulting in difficulties with cast restorations. (a) Fracture of porcelain restorations as a result of insufficient tooth reduction. (b) The restoration on tooth 36 is perforated (arrows) as a result of insufficient occlusal reduction. (c) The preparation on tooth 22 did not create sufficient space for restorative material and the restoration was overcontoured. Recontouring the restoration resulted in 'show-through' of the opaque porcelain, leading to aesthetic failure.

opment of more optimal aesthetics, especially in the gingival embrasures, will play a significant role in the level of the finish-line placement. Deeper finish lines will be required to limit 'cervical black line' and 'black triangle' effects being created in the final restorations - in particular where significant gingival recession is present initially.

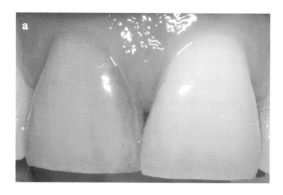

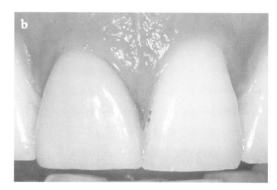

Fig 2-5 Restoration of discoloured teeth. Restoration of a darkened tooth using a combination of bleaching and an Empress porcelain laminate veneer. (a) Pre-op view. (b) Post-op view. The patient declined the option for gingival margin correction (courtesy of Dr. K O'Boyle).

Conclusion

Creation of an optimal preparation shape is the starting point in developing a closely adapted restoration, limiting dependence on the physical properties of the luting cement, while satisfying mechanical, biological and aesthetic requirements. Optimal preparation shape provides more favourable outcomes within the restoration complex.

Further Reading

Goodacre CJ, Campagni WV, Aquilino SA. Tooth preparations for complete crowns: an art form based on scientific principles. J Prosthet Dent 2001;85:363-376.

Goodacre CJ, Bernal G, Rungcharassaeng K, Kan JY. Clinical complications in fixed prosthodontics. J Prosthet Dent 2003;90:31-41.

Shillingburg HT Jr, Jacobi R, Brackett SE. Preparation modifications for damaged vital posterior teeth. Dent Clin North Am 1985;29:305–326.

Walton TR. A 10-year longitudinal study of fixed prosthodontics: clinical characteristics and outcome of single-unit metal-ceramic crowns. Int J Prosthodont 1999;12:519–526.

Chapter 3
Restorative Periodontal Interface

Aim

The aim of this chapter is to provide the practitioner with an understanding of the concept of biological width and to illustrate various soft-tissue procedures that may enhance restorative outcomes.

Outcome

Maintenance of periodontal health is a key component in successful restorative dentistry. The gingival tissues provide a background against which a prosthesis is viewed, yet they are often overlooked when restorative dental treatment is planned. Therefore designing restorations that maintain gingival health is part of the planning process. An aspect of this process, often omitted, is the prescription of surgical procedures to alter hard and soft-tissue relationships.

Biological Width

Biological width is a term used to describe the amount or extent of soft tissue between the crest of the alveolar ridge and the base of the gingival sulcus (Fig 3-1). This soft tissue is made up of the junctional epithelium and supercrestal connective tissues. Its dimension is between 2-3mm. If this dimension is not allowed for during periodontal surgical procedures or impinged upon during the placement of a restoration, adverse periodontal reactions may occur.

A common error during crown preparation is failure to allow for the papilla height resulting in the interproximal surfaces being prepared to the same level as the buccal and palatal surfaces, thus creating a subgingival finish line interproximally. This impingement is often enough to result in an inflammatory infiltrate tracking around the entire buccal surface of the tooth.

Biological width is important when crown-lengthening surgery is being considered. Prior to completion of the surgery, the dimensions of the gingival

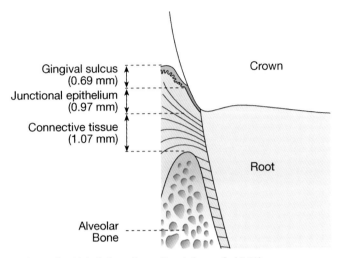

Fig 3-1 Biological width (taken from Gargiulo et al, 1961).

soft tissue should be established. It should be determined whether osseous reduction is required and if so, how much bony tissue should be removed. If this soft-tissue dimension is not allowed for when removing osseous tissue, it is possible that inadequate crown length will be achieved, necessitating corrective procedures.

At least 3mm should be allowed from above the osseous crest to the new restorative margin. Alternatively, prior to surgery, the distance from the gingival crest to the alveolar crest can be measured using a periodontal probe when the patient is anaesthetised. This dimension can then be used as a guide as to the distance from the new restorative margin to the alveolar crest.

Periodontal Restorative Interface in Restorative Dentistry

Restorative Margin Placement

The location of a restorative margin has generated much debate. Three possible options exist: supragingival, intracrevicular and subgingival (Fig 3-2).

Supragingival margin placement ensures that the junction between the restoration and the tooth is above the gingival margin. This option is the most compatible with gingival health. However, this approach can produce

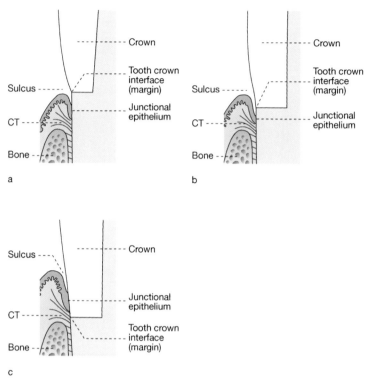

Fig 3-2 Margin placement levels. (a) Supragingival margin. (b) Intracrevicular margin. c) Subgingival margin.

suboptimal aesthetics. Where aesthetics are an issue a suitable compromise is the intracrevicular margin, placed within the gingival sulcus but not impinging on the junctional epithelium. Ideally this margin is located 0.5-1mm apical to the free gingival margin. The subgingival margin is located below the base of the gingival sulcus, impinging upon the biological width. This approach has previously been advocated to gain retention in short tooth preparations, avoid sensitivity, offer protection from caries and enhance aesthetics. Unfortunately the usual consequences of biological width invasion are inflammation, periodontal disease and recession.

Treatment of Marginal Tissues During Impression-Making

Soft-tissue management is important for optimal impression-making. Various methods have been advocated to ensure an adequate bulk of impression

material around the teeth and that the margins of preparations are visible in the impression (Fig 3-3). Three common techniques are:
- gingival curettage
- electrosurgery
- retraction materials.

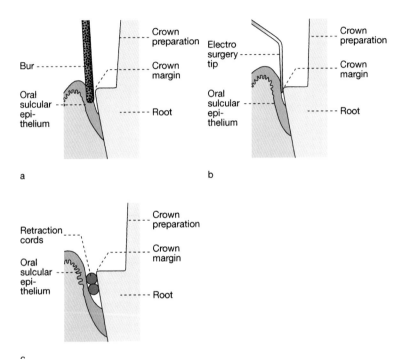

c

Fig 3-3 Methods available for gingival retraction. (a) Gingival curettage. (b) Electrosurgery. c) Retraction cord (two-cord technique demonstrated).

Gingival curettage and electrosurgery remove tissue from around the preparation margin. In gingival curettage a diamond bur is placed within the sulcus and gently moved around the crevice, removing part of the soft tissue wall. An electrosurgery unit eliminates these cells. The objective of both techniques is to produce a trough around the tooth, exposing the prepared margin for the impression.

Retraction cords displace the tissue away from the prepared margin and, if a vasoconstrictor is used, cause shrinking of the tissue due to constriction of the small blood vessels of the gingiva.

Controversy exists as to which technique is the least damaging to the gingival tissues. Even when used correctly each technique will cause a small amount of recession, usually in the order of 0.1mm. Research on all three techniques has not demonstrated superiority of one over the other two. All three are useful in selected situations. However, misapplication of any of these retraction methods will result in serious consequences, such as pain and recession. Common to each technique is the need for gentle handling of the tissue and minimal application, consistent with achieving the objective, of the retraction agent. After the impression is made the patient should be advised to rinse with chlorhexidine mouthwash to ensure optimal soft-tissue healing.

Surgical Procedures to Enhance Restorative Outcomes

Crown-Lengthening Surgery
Definition
A surgical procedure to expose tooth structure located below the gingival margin by the removal of soft tissue and bone (Fig 3-4).

Indications
Functional crown-lengthening is indicated when there is not enough tooth substance present supragingivally to allow a predictable restoration to be placed. This commonly occurs when a tooth has been fractured, worn, extensively restored or is otherwise badly deteriorated. If this situation is not treated there will be insufficient tooth substance to retain a restoration, or in order to gain preparation height the final finish line will have to be extended subgingivally, invading the biological width. It should be noted that in certain circumstances minimal biological width invasion might be acceptable as an alternative compromise to extensive surgery.

Aesthetic crown-lengthening is completed on the facial aspect to enhance the aesthetic outcome. Two commonly occurring situations where crown-lengthening may be indicated are after extensive wear and delayed passive eruption. In extensive wear cases it may be necessary to crown-lengthen, prior to fixed reconstruction, to ensure the final restorations have sufficient resistance and retention form and appear properly proportioned. Delayed passive eruption occurs when the clinical crown of a tooth has not fully erupted into the oral cavity. The gingival margin is located above the cemento-enamel junction, its usual position. This results in a 'gummy' smile, as too much gingiva is displayed. The teeth appear unaesthetic, presenting as square rather than rectangular in shape as the normally ratio of height to width is altered.

29

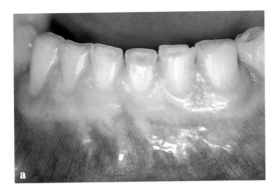

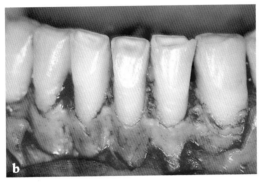

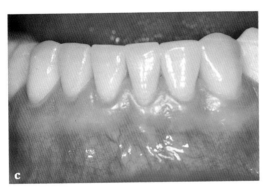

Fig 3-4 Crown lengthening. (a) Anterior mandibular sextant requiring crown lengthening prior to restoration. (b) Labial flap reflected and osseous tissue removed and recontoured. (c) Porcelain crowns placed after periodontal healing.

Assessment

Preoperative assessment is critical to the success of crown lengthening surgery. The following should be considered to ensure an optimal outcome:

- *Tooth restorability* - if extensive tooth loss has occurred, is the tooth restorable? If yes, but crown-lengthening surgery, endodontic therapy and a fixed restoration is required, a decision must be made as to whether this approach is as cost-effective and long-lasting as extraction and dental implant placement or a fixed partial denture (also known as bridgework).
- *Crown root ratio* - removal of osseous tissue will reduce tooth support, effectively decreasing root length and increasing crown length. The longer clinical crown may not be biomechanically acceptable.
- *Periodontal health* - the location of the furcation in molar teeth should be considered. If the tooth has a small root trunk, limited osseous reduction will expose the furcation. This may result in subsequent periodontal problems.
- *Aesthetics* – crown-lengthening surgery normally involves the removal of supporting tissues both from the tooth to be lengthened and from adjacent teeth. In single tooth cases, it is important to assess the impact on aesthetics of tissue removal. If the normal gingival relationship is altered, what impact will this have on the symmetry of a patient's smile? In cases where extensive wear has occurred, it is critical that the location of the incisal edge should be determined prior to prescribing surgery. It is possible that an increase in vertical dimension through the addition of restorative material to the incisal and occlusal surfaces, coupled with exposure of subgingival tooth structure, may make the final crowns appear excessively long.

Technique
- Preoperative diagnosis determines the extent of hard and soft tissue to be removed.
- Sulcular and crestal incisions are made around the necks of the teeth to be lengthened.
- If there is an abundance of keratinised tissue inverse bevel incisions are made in the gingiva to the level of the new restorative margins.
- Full-thickness muco-periosteal flaps are raised and the gingival tissues are retracted from around the teeth.
- All excess soft tissue is removed.
- The supporting bone is removed under copious saline irrigation.
- The gingiva is replaced at a lower position around the teeth.
- It is important that space is left to allow for biological width reestablishment.
- The tissues are sutured using interrupted or continuous sutures.
- A periodontal pack may be placed to ensure tissues remain at the appropriate level.

Healing

If proper technique is followed, postoperative healing will normally be uneventful. Packs and sutures are usually removed after one week. After two to three weeks, depending on initial healing, the tooth may be prepared for a provisional restoration. At this stage it is prudent to prepare the preparation short of where the definitive margin is planned. A degree of rebound of gingival tissues may occur during the healing process. Restoration placement can proceed after a minimum of six weeks. However, it may be prudent, in particular in areas of aesthetic importance, to wait for up to six months before the placement of definitive restorations.

Grafts

A complete discussion of the various soft tissue grafting techniques is beyond the scope of this text, but key indications and an assessment outline are provided for free gingival and connective tissue grafts.

Free Gingival Grafts
Definition
An autogenous graft of keratinised epithelial and connective tissue detached from its original bed and placed in a prepared recipient bed. Free gingival grafts are usually harvested from the palate (Fig 3-5).

Indications
The necessity for keratinised tissue around a tooth is a controversial subject. It was believed that, in the absence of attached keratinised tissue, recession would occur and ultimately the attachment of the tooth would be compromised. Various studies have supported or contradicted this viewpoint. The current consensus is that keratinised tissue is not required for gingival health if adequate oral hygiene is maintained. However, a keratinised graft may be indicated if:
- Adequate oral hygiene cannot be maintained.
- Recession is progressive in the presence of optimal oral hygiene.
- A tooth is to be restored and the restorative margin will be located at or close to the gingival margin.
- The presence of attached keratinised tissue facilitates the restoration of a tooth, in particular making recording impressions easier, as the marginal tissues are more easily manipulated.
- The gingiva will be subject to traumatic forces, such as those associated with a partial denture clasp.
- Orthodontic therapy is to be undertaken, and there is a risk of gingival recession.

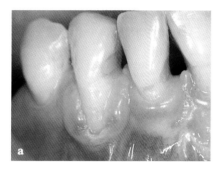

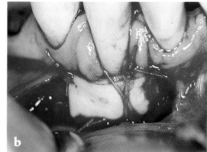

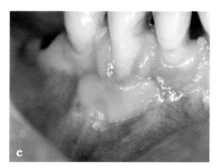

Fig 3-5 Free gingival graft. (a) Mandibular canine with minimal keratinised tissue, which has experienced progressive recession over the previous 12 months. (b) Free gingival graft, harvested from the palate, sutured in position on the facial aspect of the canine. (c) Broadband of keratinised tissue present at three months post-op. No further recession was experienced at this site.

Assessment

A number of factors should be considered prior to recommending a free gingival graft. These include:

- *Psychology of the patient* - this procedure can result in considerable postoperative discomfort. Some patients find this complication more tolerable than others. Patients who have complained on previous visits of pain from minor procedures should be educated, advised of alternative therapies and, if they decide to proceed, suitably medicated.
- *Donor site* - an adequate source of keratinised tissue is required. Patients with large palatal tori or small palates may not provide sufficient tissue.
- *Vestibular depth* - if a shallow vestibule is present it may not be possible to immobilise the graft, resulting in failure of the procedure.
- *Smoking* - patients who smoke have a greater risk of graft failure.

Connective Tissue Graft

Definition

An autogenous graft of connective tissue only, detached from its original bed and placed in a prepared recipient bed. Connective tissue grafts are usually harvested from the palate (Fig 3-6).

Indications

A connective tissue graft may be indicated in the following situations:

- Coverage of exposed root surfaces.
- Restoration of the contour of edentulous areas in preparation for a pontic, prior to the placement of a fixed partial denture.
- Augmentation of thin tissue prior to placement of a fixed restoration.
- Augmentation of sites devoid of keratinised tissue and in the aesthetic zone.
- Enhancement of the soft tissue profile around dental implants.

Assessment

The preoperative assessment for the connective tissue graft is similar to the free gingival graft. Factors to consider are:

- *Smoking* - the grafted tissue is very sensitive to the effects of cigarette smoke.
- *Anatomy* - the connective tissue graft is usually harvested from the palate between the distal surface of the canine and the mesial of the second molar. Small palates or the presence of bony tori may prevent graft harvesting.

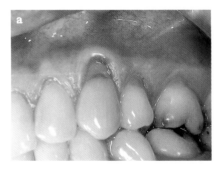
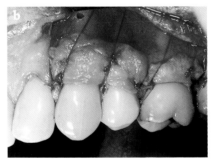
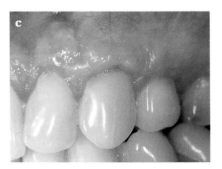

Fig 3-6 Connective tissue graft. (a) Maxillary canine with recession on the facial aspect. (b) Connective tissue graft, harvested from the palate, sutured in position. (c) Complete root coverage achieved.

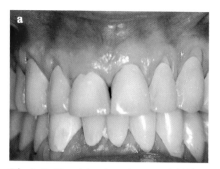 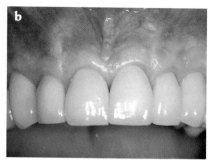

Fig 3-7 Combination therapy. (a) The maxillary left central incisor was determined to have the ideal gingival height. Root coverage was required to cover gingival recession on the facial aspects of the maxillary canines and lateral incisor teeth. Crown lengthening was required to elongate the maxillary right central incisor. (b) Gingival levels after periodontal healing and restoration of teeth.

- *Recipient site* – large recessional defects, particularly after periodontal disease, may not respond to the grafting procedure.

Conclusions

The provisions of fixed restorations without due regard for gingival tissue health will typically lead to a less than ideal prosthesis, risking biological and aesthetic failure. Appreciation of the anatomy of periodontal tissues, in particular the biological width, should enable restoration of teeth with minimal long-term trauma to the gingival tissues (Fig 3-7). In addition, complementary periodontal surgery can be used to improve the prognosis of fixed restorations by favourably altering the tooth/tissue relationship.

Further Reading

Benson BW, Bomberg TJ, Hatch RA, Hoffman W Jr. Tissue displacement methods in fixed prosthodontics. J Prosthet Dent 1986;55:175-181.

Gargiulo AW, Wentz FM, Orban BJ. Dimensions and relations of the dentogingival junction in humans. J Periodontol 1961;32:261-269.

Maynard JG Jr, Wilson RD. Physiologic dimensions of the periodontium significant to the restorative dentist. J Periodontol 1979;50:170-174.

Nevins M, Skurow HM. The intracrevicular restorative margin, the biologic width, and the maintenance of the gingival margin. Int J Periodontics Restorative Dent 1984;4:30-49.

Ramfjord SP. Periodontal considerations of operative dentistry. Oper Dent 1988;13:144-159.

Stetler KJ, Bissada NF. Significance of the width of keratinized gingiva on the periodontal status of teeth with submarginal restorations. J Periodontol 1987;58:696-700.

Wise MD. Stability of gingival crest after surgery and before anterior crown placement. J Prosthet Dent 1985;53:20-23.

Chapter 4

Provisional Restorations

Aim

This chapter aims to highlight the importance of provisional restorations in the provision of fixed prosthodontics.

Outcome

At the end of this chapter the practitioner should be familiar with the importance of provisional restorations. Of particular importance are the:
- Stabilisation and maintenance of oral health while definitive treatment is ongoing.
- Shape and form of the provisional and its aesthetic acceptability.
- Stabilisation of occlusal and proximal contacts.
- Selection of an appropriate technique.
- Impression procedure should start with the construction of a good provisional.

Introduction

The patient should be painfree and have acceptable dental aesthetics during the provisional stage of treatment. The construction of a well-fitting, smooth and highly polished, well-contoured provisional restoration with good shape and form will satisfy these requirements (Fig 4-1). The preservation of the

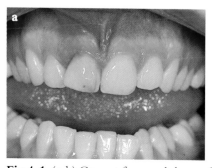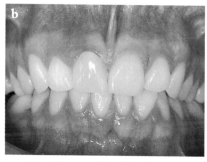

Fig 4-1 (a-b) Correct form and shape of a provisional restoration. Replacement of an unsatisfactory temporary crown with a provisional with correct shape and form is the first step in the provision of a predictable definitive restoration.

vitality of pulpal tissues and occlusal relationships are further important functions. The selection of the most appropriate provisional restoration should occur at the treatment-planning stage. After tooth reduction, protection of the preparation is required and should be considered under the headings biological, therapeutic, thermal, mechanical, aesthetic and diagnostic factors.

Biological Factors
Pulpal Health
Preserving the vitality of the dento-pulpal complex during the construction of any restoration is an important requirement. The biological integrity of the complex is maintained by careful construction of a provisional restoration so it seals the dentinal complex from the oral environment, allowing resolution of any pulpitis following tooth preparation. The damage to the pulp from exposure to microbial insult through the recently cut and open tubules must be minimised. Provisional restorations, with accurate fit and marginal adaptation, allow temporary luting agents to seal the preparation from oral fluid and bacterial ingress.

Gingival Factors
Gingival and periodontal health must be preserved. Some gingival trauma is inevitable if the finish line of the preparation is placed at or below the gingival crest and retraction cord is used during impression procedures. Rapid and complete healing of this trauma is required.

Increased awareness of gingival aesthetics increases the demand for aesthetically pleasing provisional restorations. Inadequate provisional restorations will be unsightly and compromise the restoration/periodontal relationship. To proceed with a final impression without establishing this delicate relationship is to invite aesthetic failure, which will manifest itself in exposure of the root surface when the gingival health is restored. This may not become apparent until after placement of the definitive restoration. The final shape, form and contour of the gingival margins can also be assessed in the provisional restorations.

Diagnostic-Gingival
Gingival contour can also be assessed with good provisional restorations. Provisionals may be evaluated to determine if the definitive restoration(s) may be improved by:
- extending tooth preparations
- modification of tooth length/lip relations
- changing contours and emergence profiles

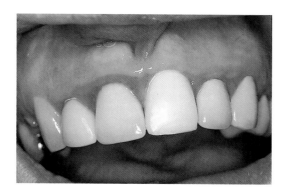

Fig 4-2 Poor gingival health secondary to iatrogenic factors. The damaging effects of previous poorly fitting or overextended restorations are initially treated with provisional restorations. However, further periodontal intervention may be required.

- altering the occlusal arrangement
- altering of the shape and form of the gingival tissues
- assessing phonetics.

Periodontal health is preserved through the creation of correct contours, embrasure spaces and the correct location and dimension of proximal contacts. The provisional restoration must not interfere with routine oral hygiene procedures and allow full plaque removal. The patient's ability to successfully remove plaque from the provisional restoration is largely dependent on the contour and surface finish of the restoration. This can be difficult to achieve, and later in the chapter consideration is given to techniques to achieve a provisional restoration with the optimal form and shape.

Existing poor periodontal health secondary to iatrogenic factors – for instance, poorly fitting existing restorations (Fig 4-2) or overextended restorations - can be improved by provisional restoration placement. If resolution is not achieved through this approach, further periodontal intervention is indicated prior to definitive treatment.

A critical test of any provisional technique is to place the cleaned provisional restoration on the die or model of the definitive tooth preparations after treatment and assess the adequacy of fit and contour.

Therapeutic

To protect pulpal vitality a multiple stage reduction of the tooth may be recommended. With the extensive tooth reduction required for metal-ceramic crowns and certain all-ceramic systems, a provisional restoration may be considered for a longer period of time to allow secondary dentine formation prior to proceeding with final tooth preparation, impression-making or final cementation. The benefit of a two-stage reduction in such a preparation of the tooth should be considered. The initial phase of the preparation would stimulate secondary formation, and continuing the preparation at a later time may allow the safe removal of the required amount of tooth. Similarly, a tooth with a minor misalignment or in a young adult might not require elective devitalisation with two-stage reduction of the tooth.

Thermal

Thermal insult to a prepared tooth may cause discomfort and add to the trauma of tooth preparation. The provisional restoration will protect the tooth from thermal insult. The materials used for provisional restorations are good thermal insulators. Good fit and adequate luting will prevent leakage, which is also required to ensure thermal protection.

During construction of a provisional restoration, the exothermic setting reaction of the material must not be allowed to provide a thermal insult to the tooth. Removing the incompletely cured restoration at an appropriate time is critical to limiting thermal insult.

Mechanical

- *Positional stability* – the position of the prepared tooth must be maintained. Good proximal and occlusal contacts will prevent migration of the tooth during the provisional period. This in turn will reduce the length of the restoration placement visit and the frequency of laboratory remakes. Low polymerisation shrinkage in the chosen material will facilitate this. A material with good wear resistance and suitable fracture resistance is also required to resist damage during functional loading.
- *Restoration strength* – the provisional restoration must have sufficient strength to resist fracture and deformation, which results in cementation failure. Resistance to deformation can be increased with polyethylene fibre ribbons or the use of a cast metal framework. Failure of the provisional restoration cemented during treatment is a source of irritation to the patient and frustration to the dentist. It can also necessitate repeat impressions and laboratory remakes.
- *Retentive nature of preparation* – the provisional also allows an assessment of the retentive potential of a tooth preparation. Using standard techniques and conventional provisional luting agents the retention should not fail. If repeated failure occurs, the resistance and retention form of the tooth

preparation or the design of the occlusal scheme may need to be improved before proceeding to the definitive restoration.

Aesthetic and Diagnostic

- *Appearance and diagnosis* – a pleasing appearance of a provisional inspires patient confidence and demonstrates the dentist's empathy. Much valuable information can be gained regarding the proposed final appearance, and this stimulates feedback from the patient. It may highlight the need for further treatment – periodontal, orthodontic or endodontic - to facilitate a particular objective. The greater the changes planned in the appearance of the anterior teeth, the more valuable the provisional restoration will be in ensuring a successful outcome.
- *Lip line* – lip function and extent of tooth display during smiling can be assessed in the absence of anaesthesia.
- *Aesthetic requirements of definitive restorative material* – measuring the thickness using an Iwanson gauge of the provisional and luting agent will allow verification that sufficient space exists for the final restoration (Fig 4-3). Adequate space is critical to facilitate good appearance.

Provisional technique

In general, the construction of a provisional is carried out directly in the mouth, using a preformed mould, which is relined. Indirect techniques are usually indicated when a patient requires provisional restorations for an extended period of time. Such patients will also require direct provisionals while the indirect provisionals are being made.

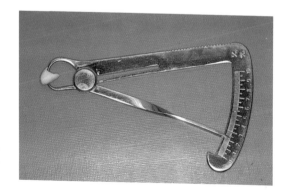

Fig 4-3 Use of an Iwanson gauge to measure the restorative space.

Classification

Can be considered by technique as outlined in Table 4-1.

Table 4-1 **Techniques for provisional construction**

Technique	Option
Indirect	Poly ('X' methacrylates) – heat or auto-polymerised Metal and acrylic resin Metal and composite resin Metal
Direct	Preformed moulds or shells 　Metal 　Polycarbonates 　Mylar tooth moulds
Combined	Laboratory fabricated shells – relined directly

Once the nature of the treatment has been determined the appropriate provisional needs to be selected. The circumstances and requirements of the provisional need to be considered in advance of tooth preparation. It is too late to consider what type of provisional restoration is indicated after the tooth has been prepared. The more complex the provisional restoration the more likely it is that an indirect or a combined direct/indirect approach will be required.

Table 4-2 **The relative complexity of provisional construction.**
Items on the upper line make for a simpler restoration and those reading from left to right are again simpler, e.g. a single anterior provisional is easier to fabricate than a single partial provisional.

Number	Location	Coverage	Vitality
Single	Anterior	Full	Non-vital
Multiple	Posterior	Partial	Vital

Provisional Technique

Direct Technique

The standard technique for the construction of provisional restorations is to select a preformed mould made from metal, polycarbonate or a clear Mylar tooth mould form. These are selected on the basis of size from a stock range. They are trimmed to fit the available space and to follow the finish line. The reline material is dispensed into the mould and seated on the lubricated tooth preparation. The reline material is allowed to achieve its initial set. The provisional is then removed from the tooth preparation and full polymerisation allowed to occur. Once set, the excess is trimmed until an accurate fit is achieved with good emergence profile. Small defects can be repaired using a beading technique or with a further local reline technique, using the provisional restoration to adapt the material to the preparation. The final shape and form is developed and the occlusion adjusted, both in maximum intercuspation and lateral excursions. This can often take more time than expected, as preformed moulds are never ideal. The restoration is then polished to achieve high lustre, ideally using pumice and a lathe wheel. This technique is considered ideal when the provisional restoration is required for a limited period only. Advantages include speed, low cost, no reliance on a laboratory and simplicity.

Indirect Technique

Laboratory-constructed provisionals have good physical properties due to the construction techniques. Heat-polymerised acrylic resin has superior physical properties to auto-polymerised acrylic resin. The quality of direct provisional restorative materials can be improved by using a pressure pot to ensure increased polymerisation. Improving the physical properties of the material results in a more durable restoration, enhanced long-term performance and wear resistance of the provisional crown (Fig 4-4). These properties are best utilised when mounted working casts and verified inter-occlusal records are used to improve the accuracy of the restorations, reducing chairside adjustment, prior to placement.

Combined Technique

The combined approach is a technique that allows the construction of a durable provisional restoration (Fig 4-5). In this technique a preliminary or a diagnostic impression is made and a cast obtained. The required shapes and forms are modelled and duplicated in dental stone. Outline tooth preparations are completed on the model. The closer these preparations are to the final preparations, the easier the intraoral reline procedures. Outline prepa-

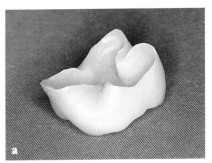
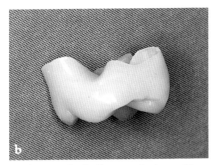

Fig 4-4 (a–b) Provisional restoration fabricated using the indirect technique. Curing of the material under pressure to increase polymerisation results in a restoration with improved physical properties. Note complex margin form.

rations should have less reduction than the anticipated final preparations to allow complete seating of the shell on the preparation prior to reline. On the prepared model the required shape and form of the provisionals are duplicated. This waxing procedure can be either a full waxing or a combination of denture tooth facings luted in position with wax. This model is then flasked, the wax is boiled off, acrylic resin is packed and the provisional

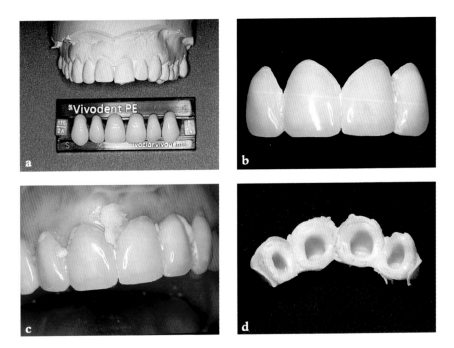

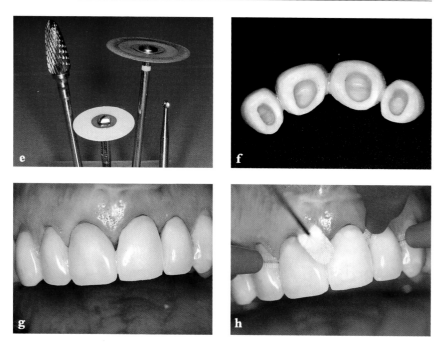

Fig 4-5 Combined technique for provisional fabrication. (a) A diagnostic cast is made and an appropriate shade and mould of denture tooth selected. (b) Labial view of linked provisionals. (c) Relining of denture teeth shells with auto-polymerising resin. (d) Relined provisionals prior to trimming. (e) Suggested armamentarium for finishing provisionals. (f, g) Completed provisionals. (h) Correct contouring and interproximal form should facilitate mechanical plaque removal.

restoration heat-polymerised. It is recovered and removed from the stone model, at which time a polymerised external laboratory fabricated shell is ready to be taken to the patient's mouth, where it will be relined using the direct technique.

The advantages of this technique are:
- Physical properties close to an indirect technique and elimination of the need for construction of direct provisionals.
- Construction of provisional restorations that are primarily heat-polymerised acrylic resin, which can be readily fitted with a small amount of auto-polymerising reline material. This reduces the amount of polymerisation shrinkage.
- Better fit and adaptation are achieved due to the reduced amount of auto-polymerising material.

45

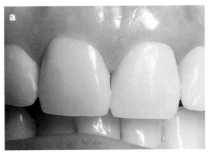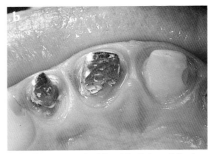

Fig 4-6 (a-b) Effect of highly polished provisionals on gingival health. Materials that are highly polished will retain less plaque, allowing the patient to maintain periodontal health during the provisional phase of treatment.

- Hard-wearing external surfaces of the restoration due to the physical properties of the external shell with good functional and occlusal stability.
- Reduced exothermic heat of polymerisation.
- Improved external surface, which will produce a higher polish and consequently will retain less plaque (Fig 4-6).

Technique Selection Factors

To help select the appropriate technique a number of factors need to be taken into consideration as shown in Table 4-3.

Table 4-3 **Provisional technique selection factors**

Construction method	Direct	Direct/ Indirect	Indirect (laboratory) acrylic	Indirect (laboratory) metal and facing
Duration of use	Short ——————————————➤ Long			
Occlusal stresses	Low ——————————————➤ High			
Length of span	Short ——————————————➤ Long			
Complexity of restoration	Simple ——————————————➤ Complex			
Aesthetic demand	Low ——————————————➤ High			
Number of teeth	Low ——————————————➤ High			

Reline Materials

The choice of the material is significant in prolonging the longevity of provisional restorations. Conventionally, the material of choice is an autopolymerising poly(acrylates) such as poly(butyl-methacrylates) or poly(methylmethacrylate). More recently bisacryl composite-based materials such as ProTemp Garant III (ESPE) have gained popularity. The relative merits of each material are presented in Table 4-4.

Table 4-4 **Main properties of materials for provisional construction**

Material	Advantages	Disadvantages	Tips for use
Poly (acrylates)	Ease of use Good flow properties Easily modified and repaired Easily trimmed and polished	Polymerisation shrinkage with an exothermic setting reaction Irritation from monomer Water sorption Dimensional stability Eugenol inhibits setting reaction	Allow surface gloss to dull before seating Remove from tooth before fully set Use of a pressure pot increases physical properties and completeness of polymerisation High lustre is easily achieved with pumice and polishing wheels Avoid eugenol-based luting agents if adjustments anticipated Reducing the amount of reline material required is the best method of ensuring success. The greater demands required of the provisional must be reflected in the materials used (methyl or butyl methacrylate)

Table 4-4 contd.

Material	Advantages	Disadvantages	Tips for use
Bisacryl Composite Resin	Systems employ an automixing cartridge systems for ease of use – mixing, dispensing and disposal Low polymerisation shrinkage Low exothermic setting reaction No exposure to monomer Possible increased flexural strength	A brittle material is produced – post-setting handling difficult The oxygen-inhibited surface layer is difficult to polish Additions and repairs are particularly difficult	Fill mould to avoid porosity or voids Remove material before fully set The use of Mylar matrices impart a smooth surface Light-curing after removal may improve physical properties and polishability Trim and polish material as for composite restorative materials Pumice and a polishing lathe produce the smoothest surface
Composite Resin	As for bisacryl composite resin with: Command set Multiple shades Additions and repairs are possible	May be difficult to remove if undercuts are present on the preparation due to reduced flexibility High viscosity and brittleness	Most readily used with a Mylar tooth form

Conclusions

This chapter discussed the requirements and functions of provisional restorations and also provided an overview of available materials and techniques. No single method provides for all clinical situations and the merits of each need to be recognised.

In summary:
- Gingival tissue health is a prerequisite for successful impression-making.
- A good provisional restoration is required for successful protection of the dental pulp and adjacent gingival tissues after preparation.
- A provisional also maintains the spatial relationships of the tooth following preparation.

Further Reading

Haselton DR, Diaz-Arnold AM, Vargas MA. Flexural strength of provisional crown and fixed partial denture resin. J Prosthet Dent 2002;87:225-228.

Koumijan JH, Nimmo A. Evaluation of fracture resistance of resins used for provisional restorations. J Prosthet Dent 1990;64:654-657.

Sen D, Goller G, Issever H. The effect of two polishing pastes on the surface roughness of bis-acryl composite and methacrylate-based resins. J Prosthet Dent 2002;88:527-553.

Young HM, Smith CT, Morton D. Comparative in vitro evaluation of two provisional restorative materials. J Prosthet Dent 2001;85:129-132.

Chapter 5
Impression-Making and Gingival Manipulation

Aim

This chapter aims to provide guidelines for making an impression in fixed prosthodontics. It will also address gingival manipulation prior to making impressions.

Outcome

At the end of this chapter the practitioner should have a knowledge of current options and materials available for soft tissue management prior to impressions, field control and impression material selection.

Tissue Preparation

Tissue Health

The health of the gingival apparatus must be carefully assessed before tooth preparation. It is important that the patient realises the importance of good oral hygiene, both for the overall health of the periodontium but specifically for a tooth treatment planned for a fixed restoration. Equally it is often necessary to remove pre-existing supra and sub-gingival calculus before preparation. A good impression becomes more achievable if the tissues are healthy before preparation. Some patients require several sessions of scaling and/or root planing, in addition to oral hygiene instruction, before fixed prosthodontic treatment. Complete healing of any treated tissues is required before preparation as the level of the gingival margin may change as inflammation resolves (Fig 5-1).

Once the gingivae are healthy they will appear pink in colour and firm without bleeding on probing or any other signs of inflammation (for instance, oedema, blue or purple discoloration) (Fig 5-2).

Location of Finish Line

Frequently tooth preparation guides are presented with diagrams showing preparation of intact teeth allowing 'perfect' preparations. Clinical experi-

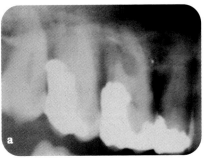
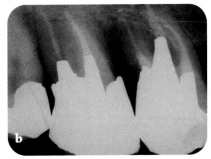

Fig 5-1 Overhang removal. a) The interproximal contour of the restorations greatly hinders hygiene procedures. b) The restorations have been replaced to reduce inflammation and simplify impression making. The final restorations have been stable for seven years.

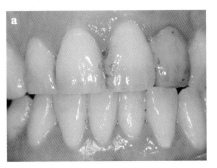
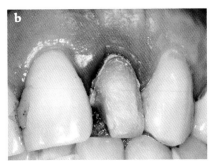

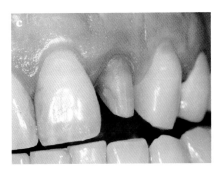

Fig 5-2a-c The need for initial periodontal therapy as an adjunct to restorative care. a) Pre-op view of tooth 22. b) Post removal of existing restoration. c) Post provisionalisation and initial periodontal therapy.

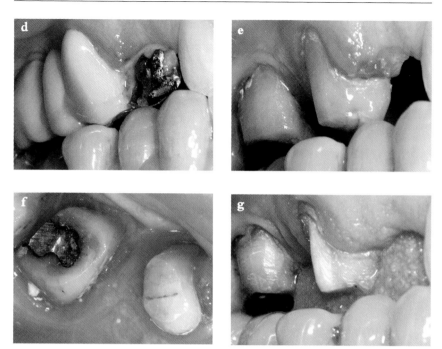

Fig 5-2d-g Note the changes in soft tissue contour. d) Pre-op view of teeth 16 and 14. (e-f) Post removal of existing restoration. (g) Post provisionalisation and initial periodontal therapy.

ence tells us that this is rarely the case; the teeth we prepare are frequently previously restored or damaged. It is important to assess the extent of the previous damage/restoration, as this will often determine the position of the final finish line and thus the margin of the restoration.

If it is decided that the damage to the tooth or the extent of the existing restoration subgingivally is likely to result in an invasion of the biological width (see Chapter 3) then preparation should not start and the tooth should be assessed for crown-lengthening surgery or orthodontic extrusion. Bitewing and periapical radiographs can be used to assess the likely position of the finish line and its proximity to the crestal bone. Following successful crown-lengthening it will be possible to prepare a finish line on the tooth so that the final margin of the restoration does not impinge into ('invade') the biological width.

The importance of this stage in impression-making is two-fold. Finish lines that invade the biological width area are:

- Invariably surrounded by inflamed tissues that make moisture control within the gingival crevice impossible.
- By definition well below the gingival level, making retraction and access for impression materials more difficult.

Often patients and practitioners are anxious to begin treatment. Ignoring the above points will inevitably lead to a poorer impression than might otherwise have been possible.

Technique

Careful preparation is helpful in preserving the condition of the gingivae. Inadvertent bur damage to the tissue is to be avoided. Several techniques exist for protecting the tissues from such damage. The placement of non-impregnated retraction cord (3/0 black suture silk is ideal) can aid visualisation of the marginal area as well as acting as a mechanical barrier to rotary instruments (Fig 5-3).

Custom hand instruments exist which may be used to retract and protect the tissues as the preparation progresses. The best insurance is the careful approach of the practitioner ensuring that the handpiece is correctly held and supported via the fingers on adjacent teeth. Also of assistance are the availability of adequate surgery lighting and use of surgical telescopes or loupes to aid proper visualisation of the operative field. The selection of an appropriate-sized bur is also important to avoid unwanted damage to the surrounding soft tissues.

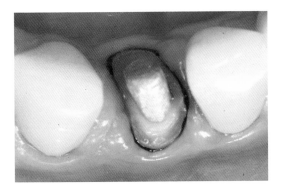

Fig 5-3 The use of 3/0 silk suture material to facilitate tooth reduction at the gingival margin (courtesy of Dr. Michael O'Sullivan).

Impression-Making

If the preoperative condition of the tissues is healthy and trauma during preparation is minimised it is possible to proceed with impression-making at the preparation appointment. In the event that impression-making is to be carried out at a later appointment, the construction of an ideal provisional crown is important. From the perspective of tissue preparation for impressions, the marginal accuracy of the provisional material, surface polish and durability of the margins are paramount. In cases where tissue health is suboptimal it is better to wait for a second appointment to make the impression and to monitor the tissue reaction to the provisional. If inflammation is still apparent in an otherwise healthy mouth, it is likely that crown-lengthening is necessary before proceeding.

Some authors recommend maintaining provisionals for an extended period of time, especially in aesthetic areas, to ensure a predictable gingival reaction. However, if the finish-line placement is at the gingival margin or supragingival and the preoperative conditions are ideal there is little reason for adverse gingival reactions, unless the tissues were traumatised during preparation or by a poorly fabricated provisional.

Gingival Displacement

Many methods have been reported for retracting tissues for impressions. These methods may be broadly classified as:
- mechanical
- mechanochemical
- rotary gingival curettage
- electrosurgical.
- surgical (see Chapter 3).

The displacement of the tissues can be described as:
- Lateral - to allow sufficient bulk of impression material to be placed between the preparation and the gingival tissues.
- Vertical - to expose 0.5mm of the tooth apical to the finish line of the preparation (Fig 5-4).

Mechanical

This class of tissue displacers physically retracts gingival tissues by means of a material placed into the gingival sulcus. The most common materials in this class are cords, strings and fibres. Black silk suture material is popular (2/0 or 3/0). A blunt instrument is used to carefully guide the cord into place

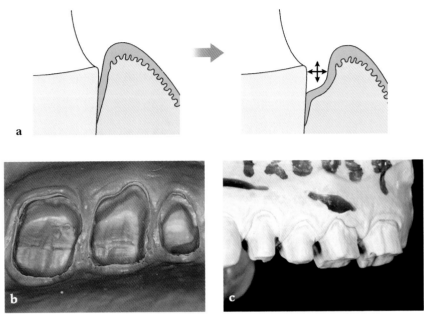

Fig 5-4 Soft tissue retraction. (a) Retraction must be considered in two planes. Extension apically is to extend the impression material beyond the finish line, while laterally is to provide a suitable bulk of material to avoid tearing. (b) Typical impression. (c) Resultant cast (courtesy of Dr. Michael O'Sullivan).

in the gingival sulcus. Specialised dental cord may be braided or knitted and comes in a variety of sizes (as well as coming pre-impregnated with chemicals). The effect of the physical positioning of the cord/string or fibre is to push the tissue gently away from the tooth, revealing the finish line. Frequently a double cord technique may be used in which the first thinner cord is placed in the sulcus and remains there throughout the impression (it must therefore not be impregnated with a haemostatic agent). The second cord is placed and then carefully removed just before the introduction of the impression material. The second cord may be impregnated, as it will not be in place long enough to cause damage. It is better to wet cord before removal in order to minimise the risk of the cord adhering to the tissues, reducing the chances of bleeding (Fig 5-5).

Further methods of tissue displacement include the use of a rubber dam for supragingival preparations or copper bands or provisional crowns to displace the tissue and deliver the impression material to a subgingival finish line.

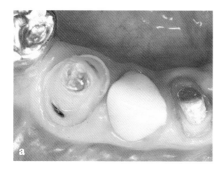

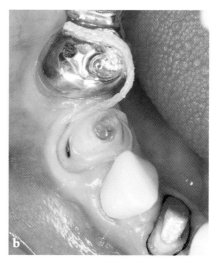

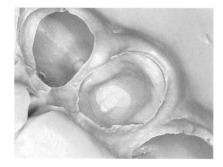

Fig 5-5 Retraction cord technique. (a) Existing restoration on tooth 43 removed and preparation completed. (b) Retraction cord in place. (c) Resultant impression (courtesy of Dr. Michael O'Sullivan).

Mechanochemical

These methods involve the use of chemicals in conjunction with mechanical retraction such as those described above. Most are used in conjunction with cord, which mechanically retracts tissues while delivering chemicals locally. Chemicals are often impregnated into the cords during manufacture but can be applied chairside by soaking the cord before use. Commonly used agents are shown in Table 5-1.

One of the main concerns driving the need for gingival retraction is to get sufficient volume of impression material in the area of the finish line and apical to it. A larger volume of impression material means less likelihood of the material tearing on removal.

Healthy gingival tissues have at least 1mm of sulcular depth accessible to impression material if the finish line is at the gingival margin. If the tear strength of the material is sufficient, the tissue is healthy and the finish line at the gingival margin, it is possible to make accurate impressions without retraction other then a gentle stream of air from a three-in-one syringe.

Table 5-1 **Common chemical agents used for mechanochemical gingival retraction**

Chemical	Tissue displacement	Haemostasis	Tissue damage	Other
Adrenaline (8%)	Good	Good	Slight	? Adverse systemic effect
Adrenaline (0.1%)	Good	Good	Slight	? Adverse systemic effect
Alum (100% potassium aluminium sulphate)	Fair	Fair	Slight	Longer safe working time. Possibly inhibits setting of polyvinyl siloxanes
Aluminium chloride (5%)	Fair	Good	Slight	Tissue damage if used for over three minutes
Ferric sulphate (13%)	Good	Good	Negligible	Temporary tissue discoloration and bad taste

Rotary Gingival Curettage

The use of diamond burs to remove gingival tissue without tooth preparation has been described. It can also be completed during tooth preparation to remove tissue in the area of the finish line. It is completed with light touch to expose subgingival finish lines. Diamond burs of appropriate size (so that one half of the bur is within tooth tissue for a chamfer preparation) may avoid removal of anything other than the lining of the sulcular tissue allowing the finish line can be prepared simultaneously. The technique allows for the placement of retraction cord without pressure. Research evidence indicates that there is less incidence of recession with rotary gingival curettage than electrosurgery. However, the latter does seem to allow a greater volume of impression material into the area of the finish line.

Electrosurgery

This technique involves the use of a passive electrode, which should be large and in contact with the patient's body, and a smaller cutting electrode that is used by the practitioner to remove tissue. The large passive electrode dissipates energy around the body, while the small one concentrates the energy in the adjacent tissues as heat to vaporise unwanted tissue (Fig 5-6). The electrode itself does not get hot. Different effects will be seen with different waveforms:

- fully rectified, non-filtered
- fully rectified, filtered
- partially rectified.

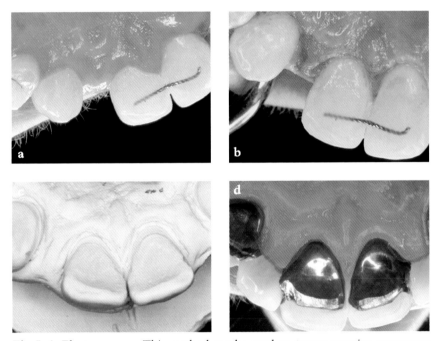

Fig 5-6 Electrosurgery. This method can be used to expose margins or remove excess tissue. (a) Teeth 23 and 21 post orthodontic treatment prior to provision of a resin- bonded fixed partial denture. (b) Electrosurgical removal of palatal gingival tissue. (c) Master cast showing additional tooth surface available for bonding. (d) Definitive restorations eighteen months after prosthesis placement (courtesy Dr. R Gerard Cleary).

Partially rectified waveform cuts poorly and is used only for haemostasis. Both of the fully rectified waveforms (filtered and non-filtered) will cut cleanly, providing good haemostasis. The effects of either of these waveforms can be summarised as follows:

- Neither heals as well as an incision with a scalpel.
- Filtered waveform has better early healing than non-filtered.
- After two weeks there is no difference – scalpel, filtered or non-filtered.

Tissue removal is accomplished with careful clean strokes of the smallest electrode. An electrode speed of no less than 1mm per second is recommended. Contact with bone, root surface and metallic restorations must be avoided. These could cause bone necrosis, prevent reattachment of connective tissue and pulpal necrosis respectively.

Electrosurgery should never be used where there are dental implants, as contact will cause fixture loss. When using a needlepoint electrode it is advisable to wait eight to ten seconds before making a second cut in the same area. This allows for heat dissipation. If a loop electrode is used one should wait 15 seconds.

The practitioner should expect 0.1mm of gingival recession following correct use of electrosurgery for tissue retraction.

In the anterior region, where aesthetics are of particular concern, electrosurgery and indeed rotary gingival curettage should be used with great care and may be contraindicated if the tissue is thin.

Haemostatic Agents
Several haemostatic agents have been mentioned earlier in Table 5-1 with regard to their use in displacing tissue. They can be divided into:

- pre-impregnated cords
- independent solutions.

Adrenaline acts as a vasoconstrictor and, in high concentrations, can be absorbed into the blood stream, leading to unwanted systemic side-effects. For susceptible patients it is therefore essential that inflammation and the potential for haemorrhage be minimised. In less than optimal conditions another chemical should be considered. Alum, aluminium chloride and aluminium sulphate act as astringents (precipitating protein to prevent plasma proteins moving out of capillaries). Any agent with greater than 5% aluminium chloride can cause tissue damage; even 5% aluminium chloride should be in contact with the tissues for no longer than three minutes. Alum and aluminium chloride have little or no systemic effects, as they have low cell permeability.

Field Control
In addition to controlling crevicular fluids and soft tissues adjacent to the preparation, it is also necessary to control the oral environment to achieve adequate impressions. Good teamwork between the clinician and dental nurse are essential to facilitate seamless presentation of the impression material to the mouth. The majority of impression materials are hydrophobic, meaning that the impression area must be dry when placing the material. A combination of properly preparing the patient by explaining the procedure, optimal patient and operator positioning, visibility, high-volume suction and a contaminant-free three-in-one syringe is required to dry the area.

One should explain the procedure carefully so the patient understands his or her role. With maxillary impressions some patients report being overcome by a powerful gag reflex. The most reliable method is nasal breathing. Having the patient breathe through the nose with the mouth open moves the tongue distally and upwards to form a seal with the soft palate, preventing contact with the pharynx around the soft palate where the gag reflex is situated. It is prudent to practise with an empty tray in a widely open mouth.

While many patients prefer to be sitting up for maxillary impressions, it is possible to make a maxillary impression while the patient is supine. Controlled breathing is a prerequisite. The main advantage of a supine patient is that the clinician can directly view the area. Thus the area can be dried and kept dry while the tray is loaded and inserted.

Mandibular arch impressions usually do not tend to stimulate a gag reflex. For mandibular impressions lighting and direct vision are more favourable with the patient sitting up; however, many clinicians opt to keep the patient supine for ergonomic reasons. Before positioning the patient it is prudent to allow him or her to rinse so to remove any viscous saliva or loose debris. The three-in-one syringe should be capable of supplying a pure air jet without oil or water contamination.

Impression Trays and Materials

Impression trays can be stock (metal or plastic) or custom-made. Clinical experience suggests that stock trays are suitable for most clinical situations. Custom trays are advisable in the following instances:
- Making an impression of the most distal tooth in a dental arch.
- Where the arch form does not conform to the dimensions of the stock tray.

- Multiple preparations.
- Long tooth-span fixed partial dentures.

Individual preference dictates the impression tray type but all need to be rigid, conform to the dental arch and include all the teeth in the arch.

One should select the most appropriate material for each case. Materials can be used successfully as a one- or two-stage technique (heavy body or putty material supporting a low-viscosity wash material). However, to prevent distortion, it is essential to avoid plastic stock trays with the two-stage technique.

While it is cost-effective to stock only one impression material, there are times when having an alternative can be advantageous. The most commonly used types of impression material for fixed prosthodontics are:
- polyvinyl siloxane
- polyether.

There is very little significant difference between materials in terms of accuracy. Table 5-2 lists the main features of the most commonly used materials.

Table 5-2 **Principal properties of commonly used impression materials**

	Polyvinyl siloxane	Polyether
Dimensional accuracy	+++	+++
Hydrophilic	--	-
Dimensional stability	+++	++
Multiple pours	+++	+++
Tear strength	+++	+++
Plastic deformation	+++	+++
Taste	+	+
Odour	+	+
Shelf life	++	++
Custom tray	No	Yes
Cost	High	High
Other	Setting may be hindered by contamination from dental gloves	Fast setting, may not be suitable for multiple preparations

Conclusion

Control and retraction of gingival tissue to place an adequate bulk of impression material correctly to capture the finish line of a preparation is essential for accurate dies. A range of materials and methods are available for this purpose. No one method satisfies all clinical requirements, and an understanding of the merits of each technique and method is required to optimise the properties of current impression materials.

Further Reading

Donovan TE, Gandara BK, Nemetz H. Review and survey of medicaments used with gingival retraction cords. J Prosthet Dent 1985;53:525-531.

Idris B, Houston F, Claffey N. Comparison of the dimensional accuracy of one- and two-step techniques with the use of putty/wash addition silicone impression materials. J Prosthet Dent 1995;74:535-541.

Kellam SA, Smith JR, Scheffel SJ. Epinephrine absorption from commercial gingival retraction cords in clinical patients. J Prosthet Dent 1992;68:761-765.

Krejci RF, Kalkwarf KL, Krause-Hohenstein U. Electrosurgery - a biological approach. J Clin Periodontol 1987;14:557-563.

Thongthammachat S, Moore BK, Barco MT, et al. Dimensional accuracy of dental casts: influence of tray material, impression material, and time. J Prosthodont 2002;11:98-108.

Wassell RW, Barker D, Walls AW. Crowns and other extra-coronal restorations: impression materials and technique. Br Dent J 2002;192:679-684, 687-690.

Chapter 6

Clinical Maxillomandibular Relationships and Dental Articulators

Aim

The aim of this chapter is to demonstrate that clinical maxillomandibular relationships are an important feature in the management of dental patients.

Outcome

This chapter reviews the principles and materials for recording maxillomandibular relationships and provides a guide for the selection, use and limitations of different dental articulator types in fixed prosthodontics.

Maxillomandibular Relationship Records

Mandibular reference positions are positions with which other mandibular positions can be compared. Two reference positions are commonly used in prosthodontics: the maximum intercusping position (MIP), and centric maxillomandibular relation (CMMR).

Maximum Intercusping Position

This is the position of the dentition, or the mandible, at maximum interdigitation of the dentition. If the existing MIP is satisfactory and only local changes are being planned – for example, single unit restorations or one short-span fixed partial denture (less than 4 units) – then it is the treatment position of choice.

Criteria for an acceptable MIP include:
- *Comfort* - if the existing intercusping position is not comfortable in normal function because of muscle dysfunction, joint derangement or a combination of the two it may be necessary to consider a new mandibular position and MIP, following assessment and trial, as part of the overall management of the patient.
- *Appearance* - the MIP should be compatible with optimal appearance. Excessive wear, tooth loss or migration, arch asymmetry, poor arch form, unsuitable occlusal plane level, loss of vertical dimension or developmental

anomalies of the dental tissues may contribute to poor appearance requiring reorganising of the MIP.
- *The quality of the end-stop* - the existing MIP should provide a definitive end-stop position for the mandible on elevation, with even, simultaneous tooth contacts on right and left sides. Normally this requires a minimum of two or three contacts (functioning units) in the premolar/molar region on both sides, with light contacts on anterior teeth. If such a position is to be recorded accurately, sufficient contacts must exist to allow steady, unambiguous interdigitation of the casts.

Centric Maxillomandibular Relation

This position is independent of tooth contact. The only movement that occurs in the CMMR is a hinge-like movement in the inferior compartments of the articulation. CMMR has been advocated as a treatment position when the current MIP is not available or suitable – for example, an inadequate end-stop or advanced tooth-wear making precise identification of the position unclear. There is much empirical support for the use of this position. This position is difficult to identify as it is determined by a normal arrangement of anatomical structures of the craniomandibular articulation (CMA) and these cannot be seen by the clinician. This is particularly so where a degree of mandibular muscle dysfunction exists.

Clinical Techniques to Record Mandibular Relationships

Clinical recording of maxillomandibular relationships is divided into two phases:
- Setting the maxillary cast in correct relationship to the transverse axis of the articulator.
- Setting the mandibular cast in correct relationship to the transverse axis of the articulator.

Dental Articulators

The function of dental articulators is to hold casts of the maxilla or mandible to simulate clinical positional relationships and relationships during some mandibular movements. A wide range of articulators is available, each with its own indications and limitations. The main features of each type are presented.

Simple Hinge Articulators

These instruments are limited to turning around a transverse horizontal axis (Fig 6-1). Casts are placed arbitrarily between upper and lower arms and usually are incorrectly related to the hinging axis in the three planes of space (Fig 6-2). There is no provision to use a transfer bow and, as a consequence, no capability to simulate protrusive or lateral movements.

Casts must be set in simple hinge articulators at precisely the occlusal relationship at which they are to be used. If the vertical relationship of the casts is changed after mounting they will move on a radius which is too short, and a discrepancy in the horizontal plane between the cast relationship and the intra-oral relationship of the tooth surfaces will probably result.

If it is desired to increase the occlusal vertical dimension a new clinical record at precisely the required OVD must be made and the lower cast reset with the new record.

A restoration constructed on casts placed accurately in a simple hinging instrument in MIP can have accurate occlusal contact, but deflective cusp

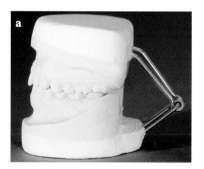
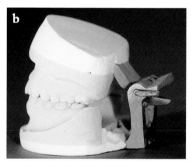
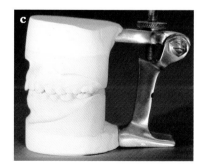

Fig 6-1 Examples of simple hinge dental articulators. The orientation and distances of casts to the axis are incorrect in most cases. The articulators on the right side have screws that stop the upward movement of the lower frame.

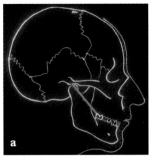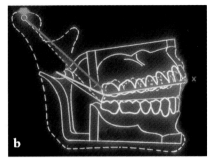

Fig 6-2 Pathways with different radii. (a) In a patient, the radius from transverse horizontal 'axis' to tooth tip is in the region of 65mm (red line). On the simple hinge articulator the radius from hinge to tooth tip is in the region of 40mm (yellow line). (b) A discrepancy will develop when the moving point is on different red and yellow radii. A linear distance between occluding points in horizontal plane will develop after a short hinging movement – for instance, level X.

collisions on gliding-contact movements may occur, as movement paths to and from MIP cannot be assessed. The restoration will have to be checked and corrected for these errors in the clinic, even though the MIP supporting contacts are satisfactory. This can be time-consuming, and the subtractive corrections may weaken the restoration or change its appearance. The adjusted surfaces must be repolished. Failure to correct deflective contacts on the restoration predispose to horizontal shear stresses that are unfavourable to porcelain restorations and luting materials.

The limitations of simple hinge articulators preclude their use in assessment of occlusal relationships and treatment planning. Hand-held casts will give the same, or more, information.

Plane-Line Articulators

Plane-line instruments can make a hinging movement and restricted attempts at mandibular gliding-contact movements (Fig 6-3). Many of the plane-line devices will not accept a transfer bow. If the right or left side of the moving axle is held in its basic position, a pivot is created, and moving the other side can simulate a lateral movement. The angulation of the fixed track is usually about 30–40 degrees to the horizontal plane. This may or may not correspond with the posterior guidance in the CMA of the patient. The distance between the pivot centres on right and left sides of most of these articulators is probably too small (range 7-10cm for a sample from four

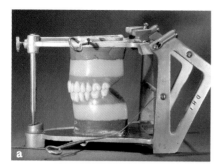
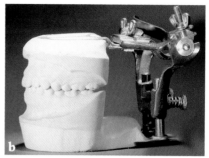
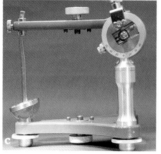
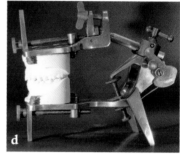

Fig 6-3 Examples of plane line articulators. (a) The rational (freeplane) articulator has a facility to use a transfer bow of the facebow type. A short slot at the top of each posterior upright provides straight-line posterior guidance. The pin anteriorly stops the vertical upward movement of the lower frame and has a very shallow fixed guidance. (b) A plane line articulator. The vertical height and position of the maxillary frame can be adjusted. A transfer bow of the facebow type can be used. The vertical upward movement is stopped on a screw posteriorly. (c) The Dentatus ARL model. The posterior guides are the ball and straight track variety. An axle through the spheres in the tracks represents the transverse horizontal axis and can move laterally. The latter facility provides limited capability to imitate progressive mandibular lateral translation. The incline of the track can be varied in sagittal and frontal planes and set to static records made with the mandible bilaterally protruded. Transfer-bow records of the facebow type made to arbitrary and kinematically-located axes can be used. These, and the similar Hanau models, are usually used as common plane line articulators without adjusting the guidances from the default positions but with the casts mounted using a transfer bow. (d) The Galetti plasterless articulator. The casts are clamped to the frames by a screw/claw mechanism. Adjustable joints on the maxillary frame allow the maxillary cast to be fitted to the mandibular cast or an interocclusal record. The vertical movement of the lower frame is stopped on a screw posteriorly. There are plane line guidances posteriorly. Usually the distance of the casts from the axes of the articulator is too great, and the casts are unlikely to be oriented suitably to the axes in any plane.

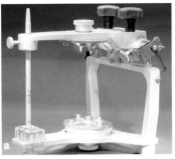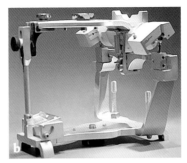

Fig 6-4 Semi adjustable articulators. (a) The Whipmix model 2240 dental articulator presents posterior guides with fixed curves (radius 19 mm) and variable inclinations in the sagittal plane to represent the articular eminences, fixed medial wall with angle of 7 degrees to sagittal plane, representing progressive mandibular lateral translation and a facility for accommodation of immediate mandibular lateral translation. (b) Denar mark II model has a mechanically adjustable anterior guide. The anterior stop pin is curved on the radius from the transverse axis to the pin, so the pin remains at the same point on the stop/guide, as the distance between the frames is varied over 5-10mm in the basic position. The posterior guides are straight rather than curved, and the 'inter-condylar' width can be set at three different positions.

manufacturers). These errors will be compounded by failure to orient the casts to the articulator axes/pivots with a transfer bow.

Hence, the plane-line articulator is not any more useful than the simple hinge articulator, unless it allows transfer-bow mounting. The transfer-bow mounting would enable small variations in occlusal vertical dimension of the mounted casts to be made without marked error in the three-dimensional relationships. The fixed tracks will allow approximate simulation of the subject's condylar guidance only by accident. Clearly, attempting to arrange group function or balanced occlusions with instruments in this group - including the Dentatus/Hanau types - is difficult, since it could rarely resemble the *in vivo* conditions.

The limitations of plane-line articulators preclude their use for prosthodontic assessment of occlusal relationships and treatment planning.

Adjustable Articulators

The group name derives from the presence of adjustable mechanical guidances posteriorly and anteriorly on these devices (Fig 6-4). Adjustable articulators can perform hinging movements in the vertical plane about a transverse horizontal axis posteriorly. A pin at the anterior end of the upper or lower frame is used to stop the upward hinging movement of the lower frame, to make measurements, and to customise anterior guidance. The posterior guidances are usually curved, and the inclination of the curvature can be varied in the saggital perspective. The distance between the condylar elements is usually fixed at the distance estimated for a random selection of subjects (for instance, 110mm). They allow the casts to be mounted with a customised transfer bow set to an arbitrary transverse horizontal axis, and most have the additional armamentarium to enable the transfer of a kinematically located axis. Within these limitations, adjustable articulators can be programmed to approximately simulate the mechanical effect of the craniomandibular articulation. The majority allow customised anterior guidance to be set by the anterior pin and the block/table/guide, against which it stops the upward hinging movement. Adjustable articulators can simulate the basic reference positions (MIP, CMMR) with accuracy, and most can be adjusted to simulate protrusive and lateral tooth-contact movements of the mandible with acceptable degrees of accuracy over 3-4mm for most dentate subjects.

This category is subdivided into semi-adjustable and 'fully' adjustable instruments. The two groups differ only in their capability to simulate the gliding contact movements of the mandible.

Semi-Adjustable Instruments

The maxillary cast is mounted with a transfer bow following the manufacturer's instructions for the setting of the upper frame of the articulator.

The posterior guidances of these articulators can be adjusted to improve the simulation of gliding-contact movements by means of:
- Static interocclusal records with the mandible in lateral or protrusive positions.
- Graphic tracings, made in the saggital plane, of the anterior translation of the transverse horizontal axis during anterior or direct lateral movements. The tracings are interpreted using a template designed by the manufacturer to calculate the inclinations of the condylar guides, which approximate the in vivo guidances of the CMA.

The simulation of craniomandibular translation from one point to another, in some of this group of articulators, is along straight guides rather than along slight curves as in the CMA. If a curved surface is incorporated in the condylar mechanism the curvature is usually not variable, but its angulation to the horizontal plane is variable in the saggital perspective.

Some semi-adjustable articulators have a limited intercondylar width adjustability, and this should favour better simulation of lateral movements, while others, especially those of the sphere and straight track (non-arcon) design, do not accommodate mandibular lateral translation very well. This can mean that they will not accept static lateral interocclusal records to set the condylar guide angulation. Graphic tracings may be used to set the inclination of the guides in these circumstances.

Semi-adjustable instruments enable casts to be mounted to assess or reconstruct the MIP. In addition they enable satisfactory simulation of the protrusive and lateral movements, in particular:
• when anterior guidance is present or being developed
• for analysis of occlusions
• treatment planning
• construction of prostheses.

They are also suitable for remount procedures to correct processing errors in metal, porcelain or acrylic restorations.

Fully Adjustable or Highly Adjustable Articulators

'Fully' adjustable in this context means that more elaborate mechanical tracking data are used to set the posterior guidances of instruments designed on the same axial/pivot principles as 'Semi' adjustable articulators.

These articulators are rarely used in routine practice, but have a role when:
• large horizontal overlaps exist which require anterior tooth guidance
• attempting to develop group-function occlusion
• analysing some unusual occlusions that occur with skeletal and developmental anomalies.

Setting the Maxillary Cast in the Articulator

A transfer bow is a calliper-device that measures and records the three-dimensional relationship of the maxillary arch of teeth to the transverse 'axis' for mandibular hinging movements made with the mandible in a reference position. Secondary to this function the transfer-bow records the orientation of the maxillary cast to the Frankfort horizontal plane.

Table 6-1 **The main features of each articular type**

Articulator type	Advantages	Disadvantages
Simple hinge	Can simulate MIP May be suitable for single units if anterior guidance favourable	No provision for a transfer bow Hinge located too close to teeth No potential for completing movements in and out of MIP No potential to alter OVD
Plane line	Can simulate MIP and limited lateral movements along a set fixed track May have an anterior incisal pin/table assembly for creation of custom anterior guidance Allow exact identification and transfer of the transverse axis	Commonly no provision for a transfer bow Intercondylar distance small, limiting replication of lateral movements
Semi-adjustable	Accepts a transfer bow Uses an arbitrary transverse axis Can programme posterior guidance to simulate jaw movement Some have adjustable intercondylar widths	Uses average values that do not apply to all patients May be limited if no anterior guidance exists
Highly adjustable	Allow exact identification and transfer of the transverse axis Allows elaborate measurement of posterior guidances	Time-consuming both clinically and for programming the articulator Difficult to interpret Expensive

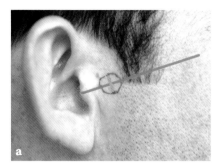

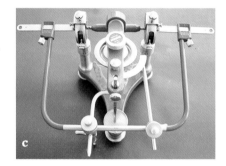

Fig 6-5 Face-bow arbitrary axis skin points and the necessity to centre the bow. (a) Beyron's arbitrary axis skin point, 13mm from posterior border of tragus on tragus – external canthus line. A circle is drawn around the points to centre the blunt end of the condylar rods of the facebow over the points. (b) At least four hands are needed to place and centre the facebow correctly. The orbital pointer is a hazard to the subject's eye. (c) The same process then has to be repeated when fitting the condylar rods to the transverse axis of the articulator to mount the cast.

Transfer bows are classified into two groups:
- Arbitrary transfer bows used to record from an arbitrarily chosen transverse axis.
- Transfer-bow to record from skin marks of an axis actually located on the patient.

Only arbitrary-type transfer bows will be discussed here. They can be subclassified into face bows (Fig 6-5) and ear bows (Figs 6-6 to 6-8).

The traditional (Snow) face-bow instrument has blunt-ended condylar rods, which are positioned over the arbitrary axis points marked on the facial skin, and an orbital pointer is usually used to approximately relate the occlusal plane to the Frankfort Plane via a third anterior point. Difficulties with face-bow instruments include the requirement for two operators and additional clinical time and these features have rendered them obsolete.

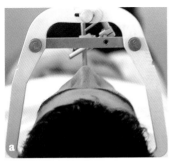
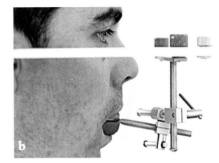

Fig 6-6 Location of the ear-bow on the patient. Recording distance and orientation of maxillary dentition to transverse 'axis' for mandibular hinging movements in the reference position. (a) The bow self-centres on the patient's head and on the articulator. Broken line = line between the machined holes in the earpieces. (b) the earpieces fit snugly in the external auditory meati. On this transfer-bow the undersurface of the side arm is the level of the Frankfort plane, and here is set level with the lowest point on the orbital rim (red dot), or a Nasion relator can be used to set the transfer-bow to this level automatically.

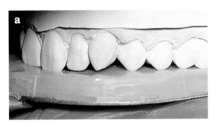
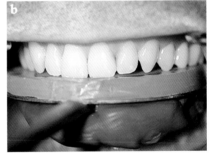

Fig 6-7 Preparation of the transfer-bow fork. (a) Transfer-bow fork with accurate shallow imprints of the maxillary teeth. Direct visual access to the incisal edges and cusp tips is required to confirm the fit of the fork indents on the teeth. (b) Impression compound is adapted to the lower surface of the fork to enable the mandibular teeth to hold the adapted fork on the dentition during the procedure.

Placing the Mandibular Cast in the Articulator

The first decision to be made when placing the mandibular cast in the articulator concerns the reference position to be used:
- The MIP reference position, based on tooth relationships, or
- A reference position based on the CMA in which tooth contact is avoided.

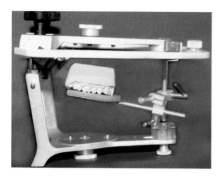

Fig 6-8 Relationship of the transfer-bow fork indents to the posterior of the ear-bow and the transverse axis of the articulator. The maxillary teeth indents in the transfer-bow fork enable the maxillary cast to be placed in correct 3D relationship to the upper frame. The anterior end of the upper frame rests on the crossbar of the transfer-bow. The Frankfort plane of the transfer bow will be parallel to the Frankfort plane of the upper articulator frame if the articulator condylar guides are set at the recommended angle for the transfer.

Mounting Casts of Dentate Arches Accurately in MIP

The maximum intercuspation of the gypsum casts will be different from that of the subject's dentition itself:

- *Dimensionally* - due to errors associated with the procedures and physical properties of the materials used for impression-making, cast construction and cast mounting.
- *Positionally* - due to variability in the way the casts can be interdigitated.
- The slightly different position of the unloaded teeth during impression-making and when loaded in occlusion.

An indexing technique for mounting the mandibular cast in MIP focuses the attention of the clinician on making the simulation as accurate as possible.

Index Method to Mount Casts in MIP

Index contacts are MIP contacts used to improve the accuracy of mounting the mandibular cast in MIP (Fig 6-9). If possible, they should be conveniently placed for visual access and testing with a feeler gauge, such as fine articulating paper (Bausch articulating paper micro-thin 40 microns, Bausch KG, Germany) or shimstock. Contacts involving the outer aspect of the mandibular buccal cusps in normal dentitions give the most favourable access.

Reference Position Based on CMA Relationships

When the reference position is identified and the patient rehearsed in the hinging movement the tooth cusps and incisal edges are used to indent an inter-occlusal recording medium. In dentate subjects the interocclusal recording medium is usually placed on the maxillary arch (± occlusal rim), with the mandibular teeth (± occlusal rim) touching the recording medium. A brittle, tough interocclusal recording material is ideal. An

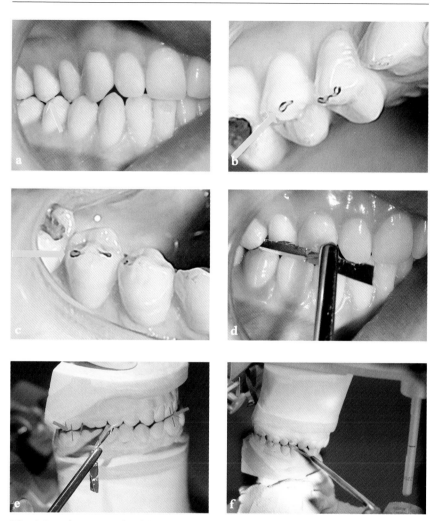

Fig 6-9 Indexing method for mounting dentate casts in MIP. (a-d) Index contacts should be conveniently placed for visual access. Contacts involving the outer aspect of the mandibular buccal cusps in normal dentitions give the most favourable access. The contacts are identified using occlusal marking paper and shimstock. (e) Shimstock is used to test for contact between the index points on the casts. When the casts are in the correct position witness lines are drawn on the facial surfaces of the maxillary and mandibular casts at three widely separated points. The witness lines are used to indicate that the casts are in the correct relationship at all times during the mounting procedure. (f) The mandibular cast is then plastered in place and index contacts re-verified with shimstock.

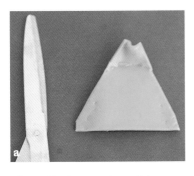

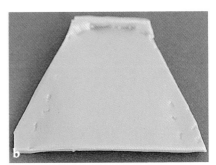

Fig 6-10 Preparation of the wax pattern. (a) Pattern with maxillary cast imprints. (b) The anterior fold-over is cut back to allow the mark on anterior tooth to be seen. (c) The trimmed pattern on the cast with good visibility of the cusp tips fitting on the wax.

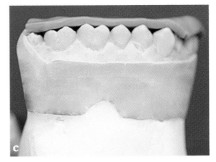

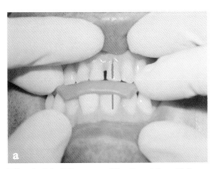

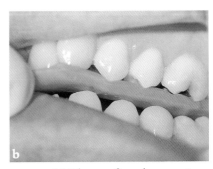

Fig 6-11 The mandibular side of the wax pattern. (a) The resoftened wax pattern is seated on the maxillary arch; the reference position is identified by palpation and the hinge movement in the reference position checked by the alignment marks. This sequence is repeated a few times from the position of maximum depression of the mandible. (b) When the clinical evidence indicates that everything is correct the patient touches the mandibular teeth into the wax and makes a few gentle tapping contacts on the wax over a movement range of about 10mm.

interocclusal pattern made with water-softened Moyco Beauty Pink, Extra Hard Wax (Moyco Corp., Delaware, USA) is used to illustrate the principles. If there are extensive edentulous spaces requiring the use of

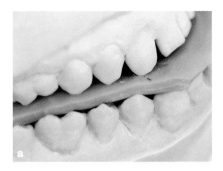

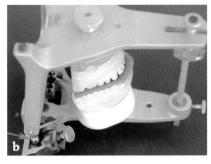

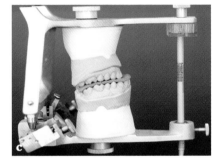

Fig 6-12 Transferring the mandibular cast to the articulator using the wax pattern. (a) The mandibular cast (top) and maxillary cast (bottom) fitted to the completed pattern. (b) The maxillary cast, the wax pattern, the mandibular cast, and the mandibular frame of the articulator, now are all correctly related to each other and to the transverse axis of the articulator. If the mandibular cast now is attached to the mandibular frame its relationship to the transverse axis and the rotation centres of the articulator is made permanent and the wax pattern can be removed. The casts in the articulator in its basic position simulate the CMMR relationship of the patient's dental arches close to tooth contact. (c) The mandibular cast fixed to the mandibular frame.

occlusal rims to support recording material with tooth indents then the use of Moyco Beauty Pink, Extra Hard recording wax might not be appropriate. If teeth are indenting recording media on occlusal rims supported only by the mucoperiosteum over residual ridge bone, then the recording medium, at the moment of indentation, should be softer than the mucoperiosteum. This is unlikely to the case with Extra Hard Moyco and a softer wax, e.g. Aluwax (Aluwax Dental Products Co., Grand Rapids, Michigan, USA) should be used instead.

Preparing the Wax Pattern (Figs 6-10 to 6-12).
A sheet of the wax is softened in a thermostatically controlled water–bath at 53°C for one minute. The wax is dried and folded without trapping air and impressed lightly on the maxillary cast, which has been soaked in clear slurry water to prevent it sticking to the wax.

The clinician confirms the presence of the mandible in the reference position and asks the patient to touch the softened wax gently with the teeth. This is repeated with gentle tapping onto the pattern. The wax can then be chilled with water or left to cool to mouth temperature before removal. The pattern is hardened by immersion in iced water.

At least three widely separated shallow (<1mm) indents are required to mount the mandibular cast. The patient should report even simultaneous contact on the pattern.

Adjusting the wax pattern, e.g. to reduce the depth of indents to ≤ 1 mm by trimming the wax with a scalpel, will tend to strain and distort it. Re-soften the pattern and re-indent it very gently on the patient's dentition. Remove the pattern and re-harden it fully in the iced water. The pattern is then seated on the mandibular cast and verified on this cast, using the same criteria as for the maxillary cast. If the cast is not being mounted immediately the pattern should be stored on the upper or lower cast in the non-freezer compartment of a domestic refrigerator.

Checking the Mounted Relationship of the Casts
Invert the articulator and replace the pattern on the maxillary cast and check the fit. If it does not fit, make a new pattern and remount the lower cast. If it does fit, raise the anterior stop pin 2mm and rotate the mandibular frame in its basic position, bringing the lower teeth towards the mandibular indents. Select a suitable anterior index indent and, using good light, touch the mandibular cast gently onto the pattern. The index tooth should go straight into the indent. If this sequence occurs the mandibular cast has been mounted as accurately as the data on the wax pattern allows.

First contact between the gypsum teeth should correspond to the first contact between the patient's teeth in CMMR. Set the anterior stop pin of the articulator at or just before the first contact to avoid damaging the teeth. The frames of the articulator should be parallel, or nearly so, at first contact.

Other methods can be used to check the repeatability of the recorded position, and the most commonly used are those that indicate and measure the position of the transverse axis of the articulator in either two or three planes of space (for example, the Whipmix Stability Check system, Denar Vericheck system or Bühners method).

In some cases it may not be possible to achieve a reproducible reference position – for instance, multiple missing teeth and advance tooth wear. The patient may need further functional assessment and management (including the use of occlusal devices) for the disorder before a repeatable reference position can be established.

Materials for Making Inter–Occlusal Records

The ideal properties of an interocclusal recording material are:

- Adequate flow in the softened state – the use of soft or flowable material is desirable, as it provides minimal resistance to mandibular elevation. Materials with poor flow properties may cause deflection of the mandible and/or intrusion of teeth during recording.
- Accuracy – the ability to produce an accurate record.
- Limited period of flow at mouth temperature followed by rapid hardening – this reduces the possibility of mandibular movement during recording and allows for a gentle tapping technique to be employed to record tooth imprints.
- Toughness – resistance to distortion when trimmed and durability to withstand repeated checking of the completed record. Excess recording material obscures direct visual assessment of the fit of cusp tips and incisal edges on the record and may prevent the cast seating fully into the record. Hence it is advantageous if the recording material can be easily trimmed.
- Low coefficient of thermal contraction – this reduces distortion of the set material as it cools from mouth to room temperature.
- Dimensional stability – resistance to distortion during storage if the record is not used immediately.

Materials

The material that most closely conforms to the above requirements is hard dental wax. Non-aqueous elastomeric impression materials (elastomers) are also used, with good clinical outcomes. Baseplate and baseplate-type waxes 'fortified' with metal particles and other materials to improve diffusivity and strength are used but are very unreliable.

Waxes
Hard Dental Wax
Some of the problems arising from the distortion of soft wax can be avoided by using a hard wax (for instance, Moyco Beauty Pink-X-Hard™). This has a higher elastic modulus when it cools from its recommended work-

ing temperature of 53°C to mouth temperature. It becomes brittle and less liable to plastic deformation as it is removed from the mouth. The brittle nature of the material resists compressive and lateral forces when manipulating casts.

Certain waxes have been designed for warm-water softening, such as Moyco Beauty Pink-X-Hard™ wax. Transition temperatures must be controlled with an accurate thermostatically controlled water bath, as the transition temperature range is narrow. Wax is a poor material in terms of both thermal conductivity (ability to conduct heat) and thermal diffusivity (ability to reach thermal uniformity). Thus, when wax is heated initially the surface temperature is higher than the centre, leading to incomplete and uneven softening. Therefore the wax should be left in water for one minute prior to use to ensure even softening of the material.

Baseplate Wax
The fact that it is an inexpensive material is its most redeeming feature. Difficulties with baseplate wax include:
- A weak intermolecular structure. As a result heating in a flame, hot air or warm water irreversibly damages the wax surface. This renders it unable to produce an accurate imprint.
- The inability to be uniformly heated in water, as its components separate and flow away.
- High-flow properties reducing the ability to verify interocclusal records or trim the record without distortion.
- A long working time. As the mandible does not hold tooth-contact positions for more than fractions of a second, slow hardening introduces inaccuracies in the record.
- Inherent distortion on removal. Baseplate wax has a low modulus of elasticity or stiffness.
- A tendency towards elastic recovery and poor dimensional stability – for instance, contraction on cooling.

Polyvinyl Siloxane Interocclusal Recording Materials

The flow properties of these materials play a major role in their successful application as high-accuracy recording materials. They are introduced into the mouth as viscous liquids with carefully adjusted flow properties for minimal resistance to mandibular elevation. The flow behaviour of the solid form is also important for an accurate record. Elastomers have a low elastic modulus (they are easily distorted) but a relatively high proportional limit (deformation tends to be elastic). The setting time of these materials is measured in minutes and during this time the mandible must remain motionless. This is usually impossible to achieve without a jig to help to keep it steady. The elastomers cannot be trimmed, so the fit of the teeth in the material cannot be checked in the clinic or the laboratory. The elastomer record cannot be replaced on the mouth to check the repeatability of the mandibular position. Elastomers in thin section tear easily. Distortion occurs on removal from the mouth. Rapid removal from the mouth from undercut areas will produce a more accurate registration with less likelihood of tearing. The coefficient for thermal expansion for elastomers, or the amount of shrinkage, is less than that for waxes.

In terms of accuracy, all of the elastomers are highly accurate, provided the proper technique is employed. Elastomers display excellent dimensional stability. A dimensional change of about -0.1% at 24 hours increasing to a maximum of -0.2% for silicone indicate the superior accuracy of these materials compared to waxes and resins. The main disadvantages of elastomers as interocclusal registration materials are:

- The inability to check the repeatability of the recorded mandibular position.
- The inability to trim the material and check the fit of the teeth on the record in the clinic or laboratory.
- Keeping the mandible steady in the unnatural CMMR position commonly requires a jig.
- The material's capacity to distort if the cast placement and mounting is not completed with care.
- The cost of the material.

Conclusion

Recording maxillomandibular relations is dependent on the correct completion of multiple stages using a selected material. No single material is suitable for all clinical situations, as each has properties that will produce recording errors. The operator can limit these properties by being aware of the properties and limitations of each material.

The choice of dental articulator depends on the complexity of the clinical situation. Accurate simulation of maxillomandibular relationships results in a final prosthesis requiring minimal chairside adjustment.

Further Reading

Craig RG, Powers JM. Restorative Dental Materials. 11th edn. St Louis: Mosby, 2002:332–340, 369–370, 392–404.

Fischman B. The rotational aspect of mandibular flexure. J Prosthet Dent 1990;64:483–485.

Gibbs CH, Lundeen HC. Jaw movements and forces during chewing and swallowing and their clinical significance. In: Lundeen HC, Gibbs CH (eds). Advances in Occlusion. Boston: John Wright, 1982:2–32.

Lund JP. Mastication and its control by the brain stem. Crit Rev Oral Biol Med 1991;2:33–64.

McDevitt WE, Brady AP, Stack JP, Hobdell MH. A magnetic resonance imaging study of centric maxillomandibular relation. Int J Prosthodont 1995;8:377–391.

McDevitt WE, Warreth AA. Occlusal contacts in maximum intercuspation in normal dentitions. J Oral Rehabil 1997;24:725–734.

Muhlemann HR. Tooth mobility: a review of clinical aspects and research findings. J Periodontol 1967;38:686–694.

Regli CP, Kelly EK. The phenomenon of decreased mandibular arch width in opening movements. J Prosthet Dent 1967;17:49–53.

Parfitt GJ. Measurement of the physiological mobility of individual teeth in an axial direction. J Dent Res 1960;39:608–618.

Chapter 7
Shade Selection in Fixed Prosthodontics

Aim

The aim of this chapter is to provide the reader with an understanding of what is colour, to explain how colour is perceived, to discuss how we communicate colour to our laboratory colleagues and to apply theory of colour science in the customisation of dental restorations.

Outcome

This chapter provides an understanding of the components and description of colour. This is related to the dental setting to improve the predictability of restoration colour in terms of how shade is recorded, communicated and improved for fixed prostheses.

Introduction

In the dark is no colour and without light colour does not exist. Seeing colour requires good light to render it correctly and to allow the eye sensor cells to function properly.

Colour

Colour is dependent on:
• The quality and type of light falling on the substance.
• What happens to the light on and within the body of the substance.
• The quality of the light transmitted, emitted or reflected back to the observing eyes.
• Interaction between the light and the central nervous system.

The perception of colour is further dependent on:
• Lighting conditions affecting the object (Fig 7-1).
• The understanding and training related to colour perception (interpretation by the human visual system) (Fig 7-2).
• The absence of colour vision anomalies.

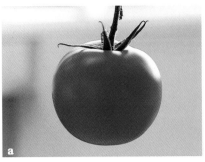
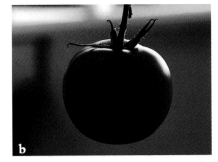

Fig 7-1 The effect of light. (a) Good lighting conditions. (b) Poor lighting conditions. Reduction in light reduces the ability to see hue and chroma.

• The object that absorbs, transmits, reflects or scatters light from the light source.

Common Lighting Errors in Colour-Recording

Daylight is considered ideal for colour assessment when the following apply:
• Middle of the day.
• Slightly overcast.
• Light coming from northerly aspect.

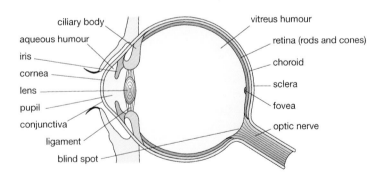

Fig 7-2 Cross-sectional line drawing of eye. There are two types of retinal sensor cell. Rod cells transmit information that gives images that are not sharply outlined and without colour. Cone cells have high power to resolve detail, giving sharply outlined images and differentiate fine gradations of colour. The highest concentration of the cone cells is in the macula/fovea area of the retina from which the rod cells are absent.

86

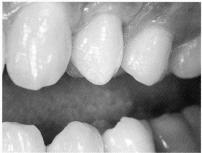

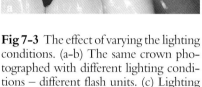

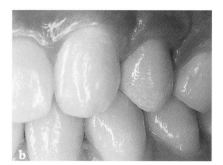

Fig 7-3 The effect of varying the lighting conditions. (a-b) The same crown photographed with different lighting conditions – different flash units. (c) Lighting conditions in an average building.

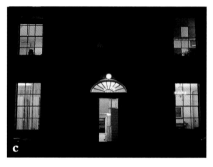

Light with these characteristics is close to the full-spectrum white light and is described as having a colour-rendering index (CRI) of 100.

Incorrect lighting conditions are present:
- Earlier-in-the-day daylight renders items bluer in appearance.
- Later in the day redder tones dominate.
- Different artificial light sources.

This, in effect, is due to a change in the wavelength of the ambient daylight (Fig 7-3). When colour comparisons are not possible with ideal daylight, artificial substitutes are required. The closer the artificial light source is to a colour-rendering index of 100, the better, with in excess of 90 being considered sufficient.

Interference from Other Colours
Pale and bright wall colourings are ideal for areas where colour selections are being made. Strong local colours project colour into the ambient light and will affect colour perception. To reduce this effect, a dedicated light source can be brought to the patient for colour selection. An example of this is the Dialite Color System (Fig 7-4). This readily portable light source illuminates the area

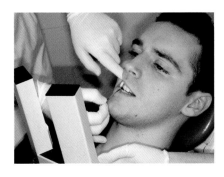

Fig 7-4 Shade-taking with a dedicated colour corrected lighting (Dialite Color System, Eickhorst, Germany).

ideally with coloured corrected light. Viewing is easily done through the arms of the light.

The Object

The object to be viewed is the tooth. The tooth needs to be easily visualised and should be at eye level, clean and moist. Teeth are brighter when dry and dessication can occur during treatment. Sufficient light is required to illuminate the tooth. The light needs to be unaffected by any strong local colours (lipstick), which are best removed. When looking at the tooth, the object should be at eye-level of the viewer, with good access to the light source.

If asked the colour of an object, the correct answer should be: 'With what light is it illuminated and who is assessing the colour?' The true colour can only be seen with a full spectrum of light. Colour and light cannot be separated.

Prescribing and Communicating Colour

Language

Descriptions of colour are very difficult and precise memory of colour fickle. In dentistry, when recording colour, comparisons are made to a standard reference such as a shade tab. To ensure accuracy in doing this it is important that each party is clear about the terms used. A useful language for colour description is derived from the Munsell Colour System. In it three terms are defined to describe colour – hue, chroma and value. Understanding each of these terms is vital in accurately communicating colour to our colleagues.

Hue

Munsell described hue as 'that quality by which we distinguish one colour family from another'. It is the name we give a group of colours red, or green or blue.

Chroma

The intensity or saturation of the colour is given the term chroma. The amount of green or red in an object can be described as stronger or weaker, deeper or more saturated. Less of a particular hue in an object is said to have low chroma and a more intense colour has a high chroma.

Value

This is the most difficult term to understand in describing colour, as it is the achromatic or colourless aspect of a colour. Munsell stated that 'it is that quality by which we distinguish a light colour from a dark one'. The range of value is from black (zero) to white (ten). The value of an object is how it matches to a series of grey or, in dentistry, to a scale of brightness to darkness. Value is considered by many to be the most important of the three dimensions of colour. With the numerical predomination of rods over cones (19:1) and their ability to function in poor and varying amounts of light, any differences in value between a tooth and a restoration will be easily noticed by the general observer and patient. Any difference will be noted as being too dark or too bright (Fig 7-5).

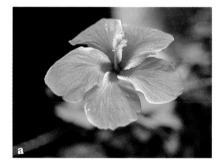

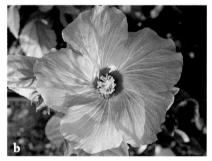

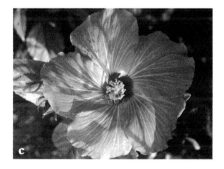

Fig 7-5 Effects of Chroma and value. (a) Flower with a red hue. (b) A similiar flower with lower chroma. The observed colour is neither as intense nor strong. (c) A value rendition of the same flower as in image (b).

Communication of Colour

The production of a satisfactory ceramic restoration is a complex matter. The task of the laboratory in producing the required colour is fraught with many difficulties. There is little chance of success if the colour selected by the clinician is not accurately communicated to the dental laboratory.

Communication can be achieved using a variety of methods:
- diagram and shade tabs
- images – photograph, transparency
- meeting the ceramist – patient and clinician
- use of multiple shade guides
- recording frequently.

Diagram and Shade Tabs

Usual practice in communicating a colour to the laboratory is to provide a line drawing of the tooth (Fig 7-6). The drawing will be annotated to describe the similarities and any differences to a recognised reference point, which is usually a shade guide. Currently the standard is the Vita Lumin shade guide. Greater detail and more precise instructions with regard to any differences between the teeth and reference guides will result in a superior restoration. Forms with line diagrams of teeth divided into segments are useful to direct the recording of any differences to the shade tab. Similarly, outlining special effects on a study model of the adjacent tooth help greatly in forming the porcelain restoration. The more information provided, the greater the potential for a better result.

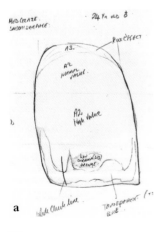

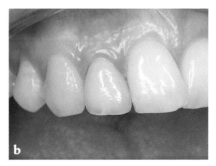

Fig 7-6 Colour communication. (a) Typical line drawing prescription for a metal-ceramic crown. (b) Metal-ceramic crown UR2 (Advanced Aesthetic Arts Dental Laboratory, Dublin).

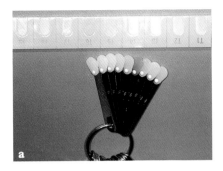

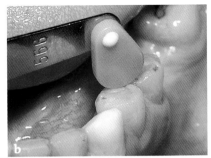

Fig 7-7 (top) Expanded shade guide for (a) enamel powders and (b) for dentine modifier (556) in-use.

Fig 7-8 (right) Shade guides showing wide range of hues and chromas

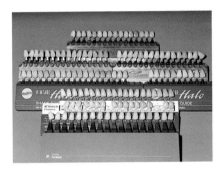

Expanded versions of the shade guide are available, in tabulated form, to help with customising any drawing (Fig 7-7). Alternative shade guides are also helpful for comparative purposes, particularly where higher chromas are seen (Fig 7-8). A definitive representation of a colour rather than an annotated line drawing facilitates the dental technician. Real comparisons of the colour, as the restoration is developed, can then be made.

Related Factors to Consider

The visual apparatus of the person recording colour must be functioning well to evaluate colour accurately and with consistency. It is important that vision is checked from time to time for visual accuracy and colour blindness. Men exhibit greater colour blindness than women. The exact mechanism of colour vision is not known but it is thought that three types of cones exist (Fig 7-2) and the colour results from the differential excitation of the cone sensors which act in an additive manner to form a colour image. They provide colour vision in a bright environment and require good levels of light to function. Photosensitive pigments in the cones are activated by light but are quickly depleted from the receptors when looking at an object. To avoid this depletion, short glances of about five seconds are recommended with similar rests between glances. Looking away to the complementary colour sensitises the eye to the colour being recorded. In the case of a tooth this is a blue medium. The acuity of colour vision is maintained with this technique. Not only is adequate light required for an object to render its full colour but to see colour correctly the eye, through the cone sensor cells, also requires good levels of light. Concentration is required to evaluate colour accurately, and fatigue will affect this. The end of a long working session without a break is not the best time to assess and match colours. For this reason, recording the shade on more than one occasion may be advisable if the operator is experiencing difficulty.

Technique for Using a Shade Guide

The current standard Vita Lumin shade guide is best used:
- By selecting the mid-range tabs of each group (A3, B3, C3, D3) and with frequent short glances noting the one that best matches to the tooth. This is, in effect, selecting the hue or the family of colour.

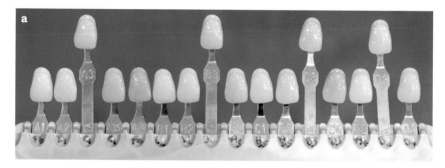

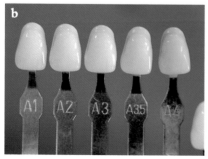 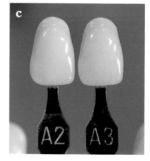

Fig 7-9 Use of Vita-Lumin shade guide. (a) Mid-range tab for each group selected for comparison with teeth. (b) A range of tabs selected – Hue selected. (c) Narrowing selection to A2 A3 section – Chroma assessment.

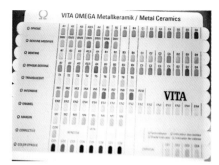

Fig 7-10 Complete expanded shade guide for Vita Omega porcelain system.

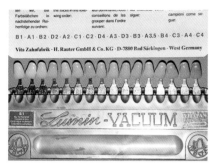

Fig 7-11 Vita–Lumin shade guide arranged from brightest to darkest or in value range.

- The other tabs in the chosen range (A2, A3, A3.5, A4) are then selected, and also by glancing the best match is selected. The intensity or saturation of the colour is recorded. The chroma is assessed (Fig 7-9).
- Colours not accurately represented by the shade tab will need the description modified to communicate those differences. The expanded shade guide or shade tabs can be used for such a purpose. Each component of a dental porcelain system, opaques, dentine, dentine modifiers and enamels can be tried against the tooth and the laboratory advised that the addition of such a modifier would produce the required colour (Fig 7-10).
- The shade guide (or more conveniently another guide) should be arranged as described by the manufacturer to represent value (Fig 7-11). The complete guide is then passed forward and back, while squinting, until one tab is found to have the same brightness as the tooth. Squinting reduces the light entering the eye. This tab is recorded as the value and noted separately.
- In assessing value with this guide, the hue of the D group is regarded as a lower-value version of the A group and the C group is a low-value equivalent of the B group.

Limitations of shade guides include:

- not constructed to match natural teeth
- often constructed from materials other than the material to which they are trying to match
- uniformity between shade guides is unpredictable
- variation from manufacturer to manufacturer
- the neck area is heavily coloured and can distract the clinician.

Colour assessment of natural teeth has proven difficult, and whether a shade guide is a true representation of the real colour of a tooth is a source of some debate. Photospectrometric studies of teeth and shade guides demonstrate great disparity between the colour range of a shade guide and the colour range of teeth. However, comparison to existing shade guides has become standard practice. Understanding the limitations of a shade guide and acknowledging the experience of our laboratory colleagues has allowed restorations to be produced whose colour matches adjacent teeth.

Improvements in the communication of colour to dental laboratories are therefore to be welcomed. Comparison to a definitive representation of a colour is more useful. The diagram has become the standard method for communicating colour information to the laboratory, and the more effort and greater detail invested in this diagram, the more satisfactory the outcome.

Photograph or Slide Images

A colour photograph or a slide transparency of the tooth with or without the closest shade tab beside it can be useful. It will not give the dental technician a true representation of the colour of the tooth or the shade tab, but it will show quite clearly differences to the shade tab and the location on the tooth of these differences. The shade tab should be in line with the tooth to be matched and held at the same orientation and distance from the camera (Fig 7-12). This technique only allows a better interpretation of the diagram sent with the image.

Currently the use of digital imaging and transmitting this through e-mail is gaining popularity. It allows immediate communication of colour to the dental laboratory. Errors in recording the image, transmitting it and differences between hardware items do not allow a direct selection of the colour by this technique but do allow for comparisons to the shade tab and localisation of differences in the colour.

Meeting the Ceramist

If it is possible for the patient and the dental laboratory personnel to meet and view the colour together this greatly enhances the ability of the dental laboratory to reproduce the colour. For geographical reasons this is not always possible, but any effort made to include the laboratory in the selection of the colour of the restoration for the patient will enhance the final product.

94

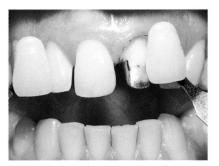

Fig 7-12 Tooth with shade tabs beside it showing differences and location of differences to the shade tabs.

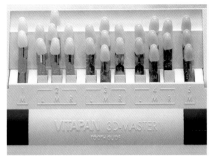

Fig 7-13 VitaPan 3D master system.

Future Developments

Future developments may include selection of colour through spectrophotometers, where the true colour of the tooth or areas on a tooth is selected. This may reduce the possibility of human interpretation and overcome some of the difficulties mentioned earlier. However, dental ceramics remains the art and science of reproducing the colour of adjacent teeth, and as long as art remains an integral part of this removing the human variation will be difficult.

A more recent and real development in dental shade-matching has been the introduction of the VitaPan 3D/Master shade guide (Fig 7-13). The significant development in this shade selection system is that the shade guide is based around value rather than hue or chroma. With this system, value is selected first, using a series of tabs from one to five, then the chroma of the tooth is selected, and finally hue. Because it is fundamentally based around the value selection it is likely that this shade selection system will become the standard in the future as the emphasis is placed on the most important aspect of shade selection. Interestingly spectrophotometric studies support the improved accuracy and coverage of this new guide.

Application of Colour Principles to Dental Porcelain

The colour theories outlined in table 7-1 can be used to develop and modify the appearance of restorations, which may assist in achieving the required result. The following discussion is confined to modifying existing restorations, as these considerations are most applicable to the clinician. Generally these modifications involve the application of external colour. Placing external colour or stain on a restoration is a dental example of subtractive colour theory. The overall colour is modified by removing some of the incident light that enters through the surface layer. The chroma is altered depending on the hue of the external colour added. Value (brightness) is always lowered, by adding an external colour layer to a ceramic restoration. The metal-ceramic crown is a good example of partitive colour theory, with the different internal coloured areas combining in a subtractive and additive manner. The light entering the restoration can be subtracted from an internal colour and the colour generated modified by light reflecting from an adjacent area.

Table 7-1 **Colour theories**

Colour Theory	What the eye "sees"	Examples
Subtractive	Light removed or subtracted Introduced "layers" reduce full spectrum End point is black	Slide projection Printing industry Colour photographs
Additive	Light added to light Sources/reflections add together – Brighter End point is white	Colour television Data projectors Stage lights
Partitive Additive-Spatial	Combination of additive and subtractive Colour (subtractive) reflected from object is added to light from adjacent object /point to create brighter additive colour	Impressionist art Metal-ceramic crown

Surface Considerations

Reflection from the porcelain surface can account for up to 5% of the incident light. How this is reflected from the restoration will determine brightness and therefore contribute to the value of the restoration. The appearance of a smooth and highly glazed surface will be considerably different from a textured and matt surface. It is important to duplicate the morphology of a surface being produced so the light reflection from the surface is similar to the adjacent surfaces (Fig 7-14), but a smooth and shiny surface will appear brighter.

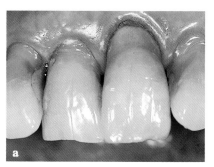 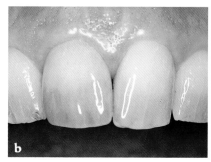

Fig 7-14 Results of effectively communicating shape, characterisation and colour to a technician. (a) An all-ceramic crown demonstrating importance of value and surface characterisation (Dr. G Cleary). (b) An all-ceramic crown with high translucency and marked incisal effects (SmileDent, Dublin).

Metal-ceramic crowns sometimes fail in colour-matching, due to a high value, particularly in the cervical area. The opaque porcelain layer on the metal may also be considered as a surface, and reflection occurs from it. The high value of many metal-ceramic restorations may be attributed to the reflection of light from the opaque layer. Glazed opaque layers will also increase the value, as more light is reflected from them. Ceramists have long advocated modifying the opaque layer with opaque colour modifiers and to develop the colour of the crown from this layer. It should be textured to reduce reflectance. It is possible that the high value could be partly attributed to additive colour theory in that the reflection from the opaque layer is acting as a source of light and adding to light reflected from the outer surface and refracted within the body of the restoration.

Altering Value and Chroma

The placing of an extrinsic colourant on the surface of the restoration will reduce the value, as it reduces the amount of light entering the restoration. When changing chroma and hue the value will be lowered and, furthermore, the restoration may react differently under different light sources. Applying surface colourants is the same as placing a filter on the surface of the restoration and will alter the amount of light entering the restoration. In turn this will affect the translucency. The restoration will be slightly more opaque using these techniques. Results from these effects are limited, as one is only capable of applying thin films of colour to the surface of the restoration. Increasing the thickness of the applied layer will cause the hue of the layer itself to become apparent, and the desired effect is lost. The colour of any restoration is best developed from within the restoration. Less addition to the surface allows for greatest stability and a more translucent and life-like appearance. If it is anticipated that the matching process is going to be difficult it is easier to reduce value and increase chroma, and any restoration should be made accordingly.

Table 7-2 **Altering value and chroma**

Increasing value	Raising value is very difficult to achieve without loss of translucency or changing chroma. The tendency is to add colours of higher value to a restoration, but this must be attempted with caution White stain is very opaque and should be used sparingly Yellow is of high value and, added to a crown of red or orange hue, will increase chroma and may increase value High-surface gloss can give an appearance of higher value due to increased reflectance
Reducing value	Brown, red and orange stains, when applied to the surface of a restoration, will reduce value but also increase chroma Reducing the surface gloss can give an appearance of lower value
Increasing chroma	Addition of the dominant hue to the surface will raise chroma without changing the hue but will reduce value A complimentary colour applied proximally creates the illusion of increased chroma and will maintain value on the body of the restoration
Reducing chroma	Difficult to achieve. Attempted by using the complementary colour on the surface of the crown to neutralise the chroma Yellow-dominant crowns require violet (B group Vita Lumin guide) Orange-dominant crowns will need blue or even green if red is dominant (A group Vita Lumin guide).

Conclusion

The creation of a restoration to match the adjacent tooth requires:

- A preparation creating sufficient space for the restorative material to achieve its potential in reproducing appearance.
- Shaping and characterising the surface to copy the adjacent tooth.
- Understanding how colour is reproduced within the restoration and accurately recording the colour of adjacent teeth.
- Understanding the visual system and how colour is perceived.
- Communication of the selected colour is vital to the process, and the greater the effort and detail afforded to this, the better the final appearance (Fig 7-14).

The restoration of a single upper central incisor to truly match the adjacent tooth is the most demanding challenge in restorative dentistry. Attention to each step and the detail of that step is vital to the outcome. We cannot hope to integrate the restoration to the adjacent teeth without understanding colour and its inter-dependence with light and how we see and record colour.

Further Reading

Munsell AH. A color notation. Baltimore, Maryland: Munsell Color Co., 1975.

Newton I. The First Book of Optics. New York: Dover Publications Inc., 1952:124-125.

Preston JD, Bergen SF. Colour science and dental art. St. Louis: Mosby, 1980:11.

Chapter 8
Evaluation of Completed Restorations

Aim

This chapter aims to provide guidelines for assessing the adequacy of a fixed prosthesis, both before the patient appointment on casts and clinically.

Outcome

The practitioner should have a systematic method for evaluating the acceptability of a completed prosthesis.

Initial Assessment

Work returning from a laboratory should be checked in advance of the patient attending. High quality laboratory work should come carefully wrapped, clean, labelled, dated, and with the original detailed prescription. The gypsum work and the prosthesis should be examined in good light and under magnification. The dies should be checked for obvious flaws, such as chips and over-trimmed finish lines. The casts should be compared to the impression, if available. The prosthesis should be checked initially on the working dies/casts.

Design of Restoration

The following questions need to be addressed when designing the restoration:
- Does the prosthesis match the prescription? Are all the requested features present?
- Are the margins as requested (for instance, porcelain shoulder or metal collar)?
- Are the occlusal surfaces as intended?
- Are the metal-ceramic junctions correctly located?
- How does the restoration compare to any diagnostic wax-up or other aids provided to the technician (Fig 8-1)?

Polish and Finish of Restoration

The following questions need to be addressed when assessing the finish of the prosthesis:

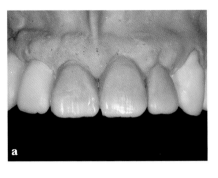

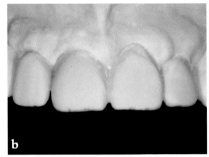

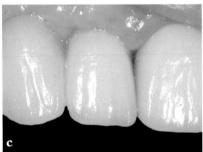

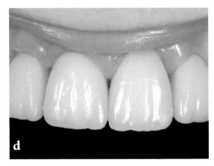

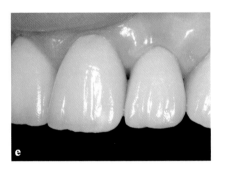

Fig 8-1 Comparison of restorations with diagnostic wax-up and other aids to verify prescription. (a) Diagnostic wax-up. (b) Study casts of acceptable provisionals. (c-e) Definitive restorations (courtesy of O'Connor-Rae Dental Ceramics, Limerick, Ireland).

- Is the metalwork well polished?
- Is the porcelain free of defects, such as dust or bubbles?
- Is the colour of the restoration as prescribed? Compare the restoration with the shade guide used for determining the original colour (Fig 8-2),
- Are the junctions (if any) between the metal and porcelain distinct and clear of overextensions?
- Surface staining should fall within expected ranges and enhance the natural appearance, rather than being a feature which tends to disfigure the surface, e.g. because of 'pooling'.

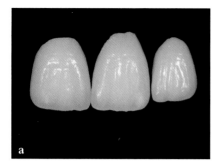

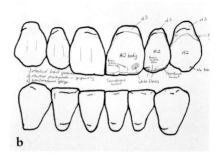

Fig 8-2 Restoration colour. The restorations (a) are compared both with the laboratory prescription (b) and shade guide used to select the tooth colour (c).

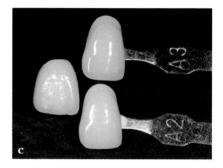

Marginal Integrity

The marginal integrity of the restoration should be visibly excellent. If necessary, the finish line is marked with a wax pencil and the casting seated to identify whether the margin extends beyond or is short of the finish line. Confirm areas of over-extension by viewing the inner surface of the prosthesis. In an area of over-extension there will be a visible 'fin' of metal near the margin. Over-extension can be removed with polishing burs under good visibility and lighting. Use of magnification loupes (x2.5) facilitates this task. Over-extended porcelain margins are more difficult to interpret and remove. Frequently the first sign of an over- extended margin is fracture of the porcelain on seating the restoration on the tooth. It is advisable to have a set of unaltered dies, frequently called primary or master dies. These should be poured first and left untouched. Their purpose is to allow assessment of laboratory work before the patient's appointment. In the case of fixed partial dentures (bridgework) a third cast should be kept as a solid cast. It is advisable to have both a solid cast and primary dies, allowing verification of the individual fit of each abutment as well as assessing the path of insertion of the prosthesis.

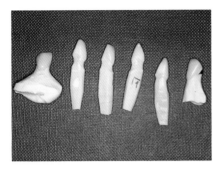

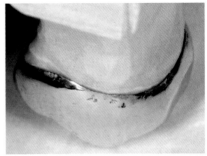

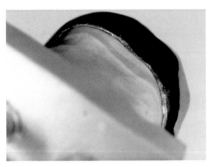

Fig 8-3 Marginal integrity. No marginal opening should be visible to the eye. Under- or over-extension can be observed by marking the finish line with a wax pencil.

A common misconception is that a prosthesis should fit tightly on its die. If it is necessary to press a prosthesis onto a die a problem exists. As the casting is seated it abrades the die stone. A good test of fit is if the prosthesis seats without pressure onto the primary dies and dislodges easily if the dies are inverted (Fig 8-3).

A range of marginal discrepancies can occur. For simplicity they can be divided into horizontal and vertical components (Fig 8-4). Table 8-1 is a guide to adjustment of marginal discrepancies.

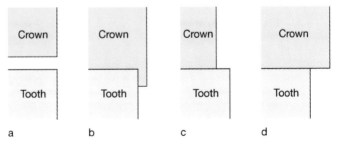

Fig 8-4 Marginal discrepancy types. (a) Vertical negative discrepancy. (b) Vertical positive discrepancy. (c) Horizontal negative and (d) horizontal positive discrepancy.

Table 8-1 **Causes and remediation of marginal discrepancies**

Discrepancy	Common causes	Remediation
Vertical negative	*If the restoration fits the unaltered master die:* • Overbuilding of the proximal contact areas at waxing stage *If the restoration does not fit the unaltered master die:* • Incorrect powder/liquid ratio of investment material, leading to inadequate expansion resulting in a smaller casting • Incorrect handling of investment during the casting process causing investment breakdown • Incomplete removal of irregularities from the intaglio of the restoration	*If the restoration fits the unaltered master die:* • Check the interproximal contacts of the casting on the solid model • If the interproximal contacts are correct then the problem originates from the impression or master cast, requiring a new impression of the preparation *If the restoration does not fit the unaltered master die:* • Examine intaglio surface of casting for irregularities under magnification and remove • Examine dies for areas of scoring or chipping and examine corresponding area of casting and adjust • Check clinically for binding between casting and tooth using a silicone or spray-type disclosing spray and relieve areas of binding • If marginal discrepancy is large or adjustment fails to close the marginal discrepancy remake master impression

Vertical positive	• Failure to read the finish line of the die correctly, extending the wax onto unprepared tooth surface or the trimmed die before casting	• Mark margin of restoration with a wax pen and adjust margin vertically under magnification
Horizontal negative	• Overtrimming of the dies horizontally causing an inaccurate finish line to which a restoration is processed • Overpolishing of the restoration after casting leading to a thinning of the metal in the marginal area	• If minor, accept or polish discrepancy on tooth • If significant, remake restoration using the same dies, if it fits clinically as it does on the dies. Use new dies if the working dies were overtrimmed
Horizontal positive	• Overbulking of wax in the marginal area in anticipation of metal loss during polishing of the casting	• Mark margin of restoration with a wax pen and adjust margin horizontally under magnification

Restoration Contours

Individual Surfaces
The primary determinants of the facial/lingual surface contours are the cusp tip placements and the location of the developmental grooves on these surfaces.

Buccal
The buccal surface should be characteristic of the tooth type and usually can be matched to the contralateral tooth. The height of contour is in the cervical third of the tooth.

Lingual
The height of contour is in the cervical third of the tooth, with the exception of mandibular premolars and molars, where it is in the middle third.

Mesial and Distal
Cast restorations should have their height of contour in the saggital plane in the incisal or occlusal third. This is to locate the proximal contact area and embrasures correctly and facilitate oral hygiene procedures. The area apical to the height of contour should be flat or slightly concave to accommodate the interdental papilla. It should never be convex, as this will render adequate hygiene difficult.

Contact Relations and Embrasures
Contacts between adjacent teeth should occur in the incisal or occlusal third in the saggital plane and in the facial third when viewed in the horizontal plane. The exception is the contact between first and second molars, where it is in the middle third when viewed from saggital and horizontal perspectives (Fig 8-5).

Four embrasures are found around the contact area. In decreasing order of size they are lingual, gingival, facial and occlusal/incisal. All surfaces should diverge from the contact area, leaving a small area of contact between the teeth, facilitating hygiene procedures. The gingival embrasure contains the interdental papilla in health.

Intra-Arch Features
Arch Form
A line through the facial cusps and incisal edges in the arch should be regular, smooth and symmetrical. The restoration should conform to the arch form where possible (contingent on opposing tooth relationship).

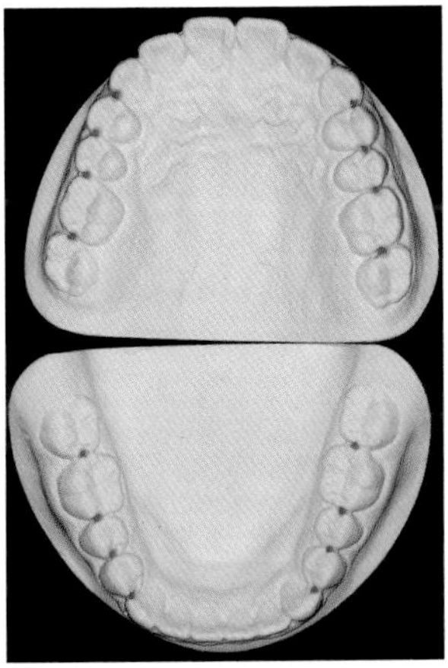

Fig 8-5 Contact points between adjacent teeth normally occur in the facial third of the tooth when viewed in the horizontal plane, except between the first and second molar teeth.

Occlusal Plane

The restoration should not cause an irregularity in the occlusal plane where possible. This is to avoid unwanted interferences in mandibular movements that cause horizontal (shear) forces to be applied to the prosthesis. Occlusal plane irregularities should be recognised at assessment and modifications incorporated into the treatment plan. These may be as simple as adjusting an overerupted tooth to the extraction of the opposing tooth.

Inter-Arch Features

MIP Contacts

The contacts should be examined using a high-quality articulating paper, such as Bausch. A variety of occlusal schemes exist, and the individual preference of the operator conveyed to the technician should be verified at this stage.

Contact should also be verified on teeth on either side of the restoration with shimstock to ensure that the restoration conforms to the occlusal scheme. If adjustment is required it can be completed before the patient appointment.

Contacts on Lateral Movements

Movements in and out of MIP should be as prescribed. This is communicated to the technician using diagnostic wax-ups, custom guide tables or casts of the provisionals with an occlusal scheme to be replicated in the definitive prosthesis. Most frequently used are incisor disclusion in protrusion and canine disclusion (rise) or group function in lateral excursions. Canine disclusion is the more popular, as it is readily achieved in most dentitions and relatively easy to adjust and verify. The role of anterior disclusion is to cause the mandible to drop during tooth-guided movements, avoiding interferences between posterior teeth.

Special consideration should be given when a guiding tooth is being restored. It is prudent to use another tooth /teeth in tooth-guided movement, if possible, to decrease the loading on the restored tooth. An example would be restoration of a maxillary canine with a post/core and crown. In this instance it may be preferable to aim for group function on that side to reduce loading on the restored tooth. Creation of group function requires planning/preparation.

Horizontal and Vertical Overlaps

The overlap relations should conform to that of the rest of the dentition and follow anatomical norms where possible. Anteriorly the vertical overlap is

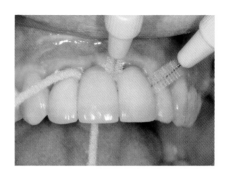

Fig 8-6 In order to maintain oral health the restoration should facilitate mechanical cleansing.

3–5mm, decreasing to 2mm at the premolars and 1mm at the molars. In the anterior area the horizontal overlap (the distance from the labial aspect of the incisal edge of a mandibular to the nearest palatal surface of a maxillary incisor) should be 0mm. This is to ensure immediate disclusion of posterior teeth during tooth-guided movements. The horizontal overlap holds the soft tissues away from the occlusal table. Absence of an overlap may predispose to cheekbiting. If the horizontal overlap is small then it should be increased or else a negative overlap created. This change in form can be assessed in the diagnostic wax-up and verified in provisional restorations before the definitive restoration.

Access for Cleaning
The design of any restoration should facilitate oral hygiene procedures (Fig 8-6). This is particularly important where complex designs, pontics or connectors exist. Sufficient space should exist for the use of oral hygiene aids, including interdental brushes and floss. Pontics and connectors should be convex in all directions to reduce plaque accumulation and facilitate cleansing.

Once these checks are complete it is possible to confirm the patient's appointment.

Clinical Assessment

Marginal Integrity
Following administration of local anaesthesia, the provisional prosthesis is removed. A slurry of pumice applied with a polishing brush/cup is best for removing residual provisional cement. Once all the residue is removed the prosthesis can be offered to the tooth. As with the primary dies, it should require little or no pressure to seat fully. If there is resistance to seating the following checks should be completed:

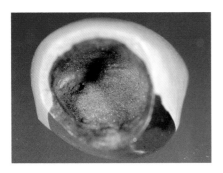

Fig 8-7 The internal surface of the casting should be free from blebs of metal and smooth.

- Re-verify that all provisional cement has been removed.
- Check the status of the proximal contacts with floss. If they are too tight, the contacts should be marked with articulating paper. The paper should be held interproximally, using a forceps (Miller), and the restoration seated. On removal of the casting the areas of heavy contact can be identified.
- Re-check the internal surface of the casting under magnification (Fig 8-7). If blebs of metal are evident they should be carefully removed using a small rose-head bur. To facilitate identification of areas that are binding the preparation a silicone gasket (FitChecker II®, GC America, Chicago, Il) or indicating spray (Arti-Spray®, Bausch KG, Germany) should be used.

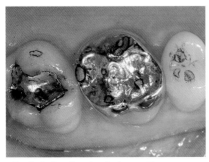
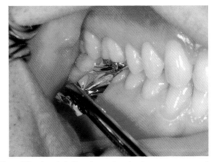

Fig 8-8 Occlusal relations. Contacts are identified with both articulating paper and shimstock.

Occlusal and Arch Relations

All relations are checked as described previously. MIP and tooth-guided contacts should be verified with articulating paper (Bausch articulating paper micro-thin 40 microns, Bausch KG, Germany) and shimstock and adjusted as required (Fig 8-8). In particular, the absence of posterior interferences on any restoration should be confirmed.

Colour-Matching

The colour of the restoration should be examined in more than one lighting condition. If modification is required the porcelain should be stripped and reapplied or, in the case of minor adjustment, surface stain may be used (see Chapter 7).

Conclusion

Many aspects of cast restorations should be verified and adjusted, if necessary, before the patient attending. This chapter proposes a rational sequence of checks to act as a guide for the practitioner when evaluating laboratory work.

Further Reading

Burch JG. Ten rules for developing crown contours in restorations. Dent Clin North Am 1971;15:611-618.

Koidis PT, Burch JG, Melfi RC. Clinical crown contours: contemporary view. J Am Dent Assoc 1987;114:792-795.

Wassell RW, Barker D, Steele JG. Crowns and other extra-coronal restorations: try-in and cementation of crowns. Br Dent J 2002;193:17-28.

Chapter 9

Selection and Use of Luting Cements: A Practical Guide

Aim

To review conventional and adhesive cementation techniques, with guidelines for appropriate cement choice and surface management of various restorative substrates.

Outcome

This chapter provides the practitioner with a framework from which to choose the optimal luting cement for each clinical situation.

Introduction

Luting agents may be described as cement used to retain custom-made prostheses or active appliances onto natural teeth or tooth analogues, such as implants. Normally luting cements are used in thin sections, with the American Dental Association specification that they should form a film thickness of 25μm or less.

Several classifications of luting cements have been used:
- water-, eugenol- or resin-based
- permanent or temporary.

Commonly used cements fall into the groups listed below:
- zinc phosphate
- glass ionomer (polyalkenoate)
- composite resin
- zinc oxide and eugenol
- compomer (polyacid modified composite resin)
- resin-modified (hybrid) glass ionomer
- zinc polycarboxylate.

Of historical interest only are materials such as black copper and silicophosphate cements.

Handling Properties

An ideal luting cement should exhibit most, if not all, of the following properties:
- Ease of proportioning/mixing.
- Long shelf life.
- Adequate working time.
- Short setting time, exhibiting a snap set.
- Flow under load of unset cement (thixotropy).
- Ease of removal of excess material.
- Insensitivity to moisture or desiccation during early stages of setting.
- Capable of light activation.
- Relatively inexpensive.

Physical Properties

- Insolubility of set cement.
- Ability to form a thin film thickness (<25mm).
- Low viscosity.
- Dimensional stability on setting, exposure to oral fluids or desiccation.
- Capable of masking tooth tissue discolouration.
- Available in several tooth shades, including clear and translucent.
- Radiopacity similar or greater than dentine.

Adhesion

- Chemical/micromechanical adhesion to tooth tissues.
- Adhesion to restorative substrates – for instance, metals, ceramics and resins.
- Compatibility with all forms of temporary luting cement.

Mechanical Properties

- Adequate mechanical properties to withstand functional and parafunctional loads. In particular, cements should exhibit high tensile strength and high modulus of elasticity (rigidity) and resistance to plastic deformation.
- Unaffected by early exposure to oral fluids.

Biological Properties

- Antimicrobial and anticariogenic.

- Stimulation of secondary dentine formation.
- Provide barrier to microleakage.
- No or minimal heat development (exotherm) on setting.
- Non-toxic, non-irritant, hypoallergenic and non-cariogenic.

At present, no single material fulfils all these requirements, and the choice of luting material largely depends on the restoration type.

Water-Based Cements

Zinc Phosphate Cement
Mizzy's Flecks Cement®, Tenacin®
Zinc phosphate is a two-component cement, consisting of fine-grained zinc oxide powder and aqueous solution of phosphoric acid. Zinc phosphate cement has a long and excellent history as a luting cement. It suffers from the common feature of high initial solubility and therefore needs a dry operating field.

Mechanical Properties
The mechanical properties of zinc phosphate are adequate, with moderate compressive but relatively low tensile strengths. The set cement is brittle. Zinc phosphate has an initially low pH and probably etches dentine and enamel, creating a mechanical interlock. This cement is opaque, and various shades are available for use with translucent ceramic restorations.

Biological Properties
It has some initial antimicrobial properties, but these are lost in the set cement. It has no anti-cariogenic properties or fluoride release. This cement has been traditionally classified as 'irritant': this is probably untrue, as it has little direct effect on pulp. The major deficiency of zinc phosphate is that the hydrogen ion removes the protective smear layer but fails to seal the opened dentinal tubules. In addition to this, it undergoes an exothermic setting reaction and has poor dimensional stability during the setting reaction. The setting shrinkage may allow ingress of oral bacteria, osmotically active molecules and liquids, all of which may cause thermal/osmotic hypersensitivity.

It is recommended that a surface sealing agent, such as cavity varnish or a resin-based sealant, be applied to the entire preparation prior to permanent cementation. It has been demonstrated that two or more layers of cavity varnish are needed to resist smear removal. Adhesive resin barriers should be applied before recording the final impression to prevent interference with restoration fit.

Physical Properties

Zinc phosphate cements exhibit high solubility. An acidic environment accelerates this breakdown, as does reduced powder-to-liquid ratio and early moisture contact. The dissolution rate of the set cement is primarily determined by the marginal gap size and consequent exposure to oral fluids. When the marginal fit is <100μm the rate of dissolution is acceptable. Zinc phosphate cements offer little or no adhesion to dental substrates, except a minor degree of mechanical interlocking.

Ease of Use

These cements should be mixed on a chilled glass slab with a flexible metal spatula. The powder should be added in small increments, a process called 'slaking', in order to increase powder content and extend the working time. The initial setting time is approximately six to eight minutes, and it is relatively easy to remove the brittle set cement.

Polycarboxylate Cement

Poly-C®, Poly-F®, Durelon®.

These cements are two component systems, consisting of zinc oxide powder and polycarboxylic (polyacrylic) acid liquid or freeze-dried anhydrous formulations. It is a white, opaque cement (due to the zinc oxide powder).

Mechanical Properties

The mechanical properties are similar to zinc phosphate, with slightly higher tensile strength.

Biological Properties

This was the first 'adhesive' cement to be developed that chemically reacts with dental hard tissues (enamel, dentine and cementum) and some metals (for instance, tin and stainless steel). This cement does not adhere chemically to noble alloys, such as gold, palladium and platinum.

The initial pH is low but rises rapidly, and the use of these cements is not associated with post-operative sensitivity: this is probably due to the good marginal seal produced and minimal dimensional change, compared with zinc phosphate. They possess little or no anti-microbial properties and have no anti-cariogenic action. No surface conditioning, other than pumice prophylaxis, is recommended prior to cementation.

Physical Properties
These opaque, white cements have reduced solubility compared with zinc phosphate. Solubility is also affected by acid environments and powder to liquid ratios (more powder, less solubility). Although adhesive to tooth structure and some metals, zinc polycarboxylates offer minimal adhesion to ceramics or resin materials.

Ease of Use
These materials proved unpopular due to their poor handling properties, particularly short working time, relatively high viscosity and adhesion to mixing/placement instruments. The development of anhydrous formulations improved these properties, but they failed to make significant inroads into clinical practice. Removal of excess cement is moderately easy, but metal instruments should be cleaned before the cement has set.

Contact with saliva or blood, before the cement has set, leads to a significant reduction in physical and mechanical properties. Use is made of this interaction, as a weakened form of polycarboxylate cement may be used as a temporary/provisional cement.

Zinc polycarboxylate is chemically adhesive to the inorganic components of enamel and dentine (higher to enamel), but the bond strengths are relatively low. The tooth surface should not be excessively dried prior to cementation.

Glass Ionomer (Glass Poly-Alkenoate) Cement
Ketac-Cem®, Aqua-Cem®
These cements are a development of zinc polycarboxylate cement. Early products, released in the 1970s, suffered from many technical problems that limited their acceptance.

They are powder/liquid systems with an acid-leachable alkali glass powder and a polycarboxylic acid liquid. The incorporation of dicarboxylic acids into the liquid (for instance, tartaric and maleic acid) led to increased rate of setting but did not significantly reduce the working time. These changes did much to popularise these cements.

When first mixed, the acid attacks the surface of the alkali glass particles, causing the release of many ions (Ca, Al, F) into the watery matrix. This early ion-rich matrix is called a 'hydrogel' and is very easily damaged by further moisture contamination or desiccation. Initial setting of the matrix is believed to be due to weak hydrogen bonding, which is gradually replaced by calcium bridging. The final metallic bridging ('maturing') of the matrix is said to be due to aluminium. This final maturation takes several days to several months. Alteration of the glass particle size modifies the rate of surface dissolution and initial setting reaction: the smaller the particles, the faster the setting time.

Mechanical Properties
Mechanical properties are reportedly similar to zinc phosphate cement. However, there is anecdotal evidence of increased clinical failure in areas of high shear stress (for instance, post and cores). Glass ionomer cements exhibit significant adhesion to tooth structure and tin-plated noble alloys. They have little or no adhesion to ceramic materials.

Biological Properties
Glass ionomers are anti-microbial and anti-cariogenic. However, the clinical evidence for this latter property is very limited.

No acid-conditioning of dentine should be carried out before placement of these luting cements (increased setting time and increased osmolarity are said to be associated post-cementation sensitivity).

The preparation should be pumiced, washed and left slightly moist. Traditional advice on drying preparation will lead to odontoblast aspiration and may increase sensitivity. Chemical adhesion to tooth structure and metals is similar to polycarboxylates, but the bond strengths usually exceed the cohesive strength of cement (cement is often left on both tooth and restoration).

Physical Properties
Glass ionomer cements are relatively opaque compared with tooth structure. They are, however, more translucent than zinc oxide based ones. This permits improved appearance with translucent ceramic restorations. They have, however, negligible adhesion to ceramics.

In order to extend the shelf life and to improve the physical properties (viscosity/flow), anhydrous forms are widely used for luting cements. The powder contains both the glass particles and freeze-dried acid: only when water is added to the powder can the acid-base reaction occur. These formulations lead to a prolonged setting time and increased osmolarity of the recently mixed cement. Early contact of the mixed cement with moisture (saliva, blood or water) leads to a very significant decrease of physical and mechanical properties. Due to the relatively slow-setting reaction, some clinicians recommend leaving some excess cement at the margins until after the cement is clinically set. It is relatively simple to remove the excess set, brittle cement. It is also recommended that the margins should be protected with either varnish or resin.

Ease of Use
All luting glass ionomer cements should be proportioned to the manufacturer's specifications and may be mixed with plastic or metal spatulae on waxed pads or glass slabs. They should be mixed rapidly, with completion of mix within 45 seconds. A useful alternative is an encapsulated formulation that standardises proportioning and mixing and reduces air entrapment.

These cements are relatively user-friendly, particularly the encapsulated formulations. They should be used only while a surface shine is present.

These cements remain useful routine cements, particularly for adhesive metallic and non-adhesive ceramic restorations. They may be unsuitable for high stress post/cores and where retention force must be maximised.

Resin-Based Cements
Crown and Bridge Metabond®, Panavia Ex®, Panavia F® and Variolink®, Calibra®, Nexus®
These materials are among the most retentive but also among the most technique-sensitive and therefore open to misuse. For use as general luting cements, resins must be either chemically (amino-peroxide or sulfinic acid) or dual activated (for instance, light and chemically activated). Many dual-cure cements are heavily reliant on the light activation, and it is unwise to rely on the chemical activation of these systems. The advantage of a dual-cure system is that the setting reaction can be accelerated, reducing the risk of moisture contamination and allowing for earlier finishing procedures.

Mechanical Properties
In general, the mechanical properties of resin cements are superior to alternative luting agents. There are, however, exceptions – such as C&B Metabond (Superbond). This cement is based on methyl methacrylate, which may be excessively flexible or undergo plastic deformation. Plastic deformation will permit movement of the restoration in relation to the underlying tooth structure.

Unless the preparation is contained within enamel (for instance, porcelain

119

laminate veneer), traditional resin cements offer little or no adhesion to tooth structure (dentine or cementum) unless a separate adhesive is used.

If adhesives are to be used on conditioned dentine, it is important that their thickness is kept to a minimum: traditional separate primer and adhesive generally should not be cured prior to seating of crowns with resin cement; otherwise it is unlikely that the crown will seat fully.

Several adhesives are not compatible with dual-cure or autocure cements. It is essential that compatibility be confirmed before cementation. The interaction has been reported between chemically or dual activated resins (using amino-peroxide activation) and simplified self-etching and all-in-one adhesive systems that contain acidic monomers. The amine is inactivated by the acidic monomer, and therefore polymerisation of the resin cement is dramatically reduced. Conventional three-step adhesives do not exhibit this adverse effect.

Physical Properties
Many, but not all, of these cements exhibit increased radio-opacity, which permits recognition of excess and aids diagnosing marginal secondary caries. Unfilled cements, such as C&B Metabond, are practically radiolucent.

Set-resin cements are virtually insoluble in oral fluids. Excess set cement is difficult to remove so the excess should be removed with a brush coated in resin, prior to setting of the cement.

Biological Properties
Many components of unset cement are regarded as either toxic or allergens. The direct effects of maximally set cement on dental pulp and gingival tissues are considered minimal. Resin composites have been shown indirectly to affect periodontal tissues by increasing plaque retention.

The release of components (eluates) from unset or set cements has potential to cause local (lichenoid/irritant) or systemic toxicity (pseudo-oestrogens). Current evidence indicates that release of eluates from set material is of short duration and little clinical significance.

Conventional resin composites have little or no inherent adhesion to dentine or cementum without the use of a dedicated adhesive system.

Ease of Use
Resin composite cements remain some of the most technique-sensitive lut-

120

ing materials. It is important to follow manufacturers' instructions carefully and to rehearse the sequence of cementation.

Moisture control is paramount for optimal adhesion and to reduce leakage/sensitivity. Cements that form a thick oxygen-inhibited layer must be used particularly carefully, as speed of set may be very rapid where the material forms a thick layer, as in cementing an intraradicular post (for instance, Panavia F/21).

Where possible, it is advisable to use adhesives that are advocated for use with resin cements from the same manufacturers. Use of self-etching primers eliminates the need for acid-conditioning ('etch') but may necessitate application of a separate adhesive stage. At least one system, Panavia F, uses a combination of liquid A and B to condition, prime and bond. The clinical evidence for superiority, or even equivalence, of self-etching primer systems is not proven at this stage. The effects of these agents on enamel and dentine are product-dependent.

Newer adhesive systems combine the primer with either the conditioner (acid etch) function or with the adhesive. This latter group require conventional acid etch of enamel and dentine (15-30s), with one or more layers of combined primer/adhesive. The mixed resin is placed in the restoration and seated without delay. The excess cement should be removed with a resin-coated brush and, if the cement is dual-cured (Variolink, Panavia 21/F or Nexus), it should be light activated.

Restorative Substrate Preparation
Ceramic Materials
In an ideal environment, the adhesion of resin-based cements to tooth structure and ceramic restorations exceeds the cohesive strength of the both materials. For bonding ceramic restorations the protocol is dependent on the type of material:
- Feldspathic porcelain (Mirage)-hydrofluoric acid.
- Leucite-reinforce feldspathic porcelain (Empress 1, OPC)-hydrofluoric acid.
- Mica glass ceramic (Dicor)-ammonium bifluoride.
- Lithium disilicate glass ceramic (Empress 2)-hydrofluoric acid.
- Alumina core ceramic (Inceram)-conventional cements.
- Sintered silica core (Procera)-conventional cements.

For the adhesive techniques the application of two layers of 'porcelain primer' (silane coupling agent) is beneficial. Each layer must be thoroughly dried before cementation.

Metallic Materials

The use of resins with noble alloy castings (gold, platinum or palladium) can be employed in a non-adhesive technique but, to maximise retention, the castings should be:

- Sandblasted internally and ultrasonically cleaned.
- Tin-plated on the internal aspects of the casting.
- Treated with an adhesion promoter, such as that in Panavia F (MDP) or C & B Metabond (4-META).
- Heat treatment to form an oxide layer.

Compomer and Novel Cements

Dyract Cem®, RelyX-Cem®

Compomers are composite resins with some of the components of glass ionomer cement, but excluding water. It is theorised that post-set absorption of water permits a delayed acid–base reaction. These materials have ease of manipulation and very low incidence of post-operative sensitivity as advantages. Their adhesion to tooth structure is questionable without etching (conditioning) and addition of a dentine bonding agent. They exhibit minimal solubility but their relative high water absorption render their use with low strength ceramic questionable and they should be avoided for this application. Even though restorative compomers tend to be single paste, light activated materials, luting cements need to be two paste systems to initiate chemical polymerisation. Although the manufacturers claim low water absorption, it would seem prudent not to use them with low strength ceramics until further evidence is available, as many hydrophilic resins demonstrate considerable expansion in the mouth.

The novel resin cement, RelyX-Cem, is an acid monomer which, when first mixed, exhibits a "self-etching" effect; the resin also acts a primer, forming an adhesive hybrid layer (resin/collagen/hydroxyapatite interdiffusion layer). The setting reaction causes a reduction in cement acidity and the manufacturers claim a glass-ionomer (acid-base) type reaction occurs. This may confer a degree of chemical adhesion to tooth structure. There is limited clinical evidence for the efficacy for this novel cement. The encapsulated version of this cement provides most consistent proportioning and mixing.

Resin-Modified Glass Ionomer Cements
Vitremer Lute®, Fuji Plus®

These materials undergo an initial polymerisation reaction similar to resin-based cement. For luting cements, the resin must undergo 'dark cure' (chemically initiated polymerisation) and is presented in powder/liquid form or encapsulated. A much-delayed acid-base (glass ionomer reaction) has also been demonstrated. The latter may account for fluoride release levels similar to conventional glass ionomers. It may also explain some adhesive properties.

Mechanical Properties
These are superior to conventional luting glass ionomers but significantly inferior to resin-based cements and compomers. Gross moisture contamination will, however, lead to marked increase in solubility and reduction in mechanical properties.

Physical Properties
A major advantage of this group is its relative intolerance, of the set cement, to moisture and desiccation, compared to conventional ionomers. It is recommended that margins are protected with varnish or low-viscosity light-activated resin.

Dental hard tissues may be conditioned with dilute organic acids (polyacrylic acid aqueous solutions of 10, 20 or 25%), applied for 10 seconds. This is washed away and the tooth surface kept slightly moist (Fuji Plus).

An alternative protocol is the use of a self-etching primer before application of the cement. The primer is not removed in this case (Vitremer Lute).

These cements are either encapsulated or hand-mixed: if hand-mixed, a plastic spatula and waxed pad are used. The cement should be completely mixed within 45 seconds and applied to the restoration. Excess cement may be left until the initial rubbery stage is reached. These cements adhere to tooth structure (micromechanical and chemical), stainless steel and tin-plated metal castings. They do not adhere to ceramic restorations and are relatively opaque, compared with resin cements.

Resin-modified glass ionomer cements absorb moisture over long periods, leading to expansion of the material. This may lead to cracking or fracture of ceramic restorations. They may, however, be used with reinforced restorations, such as Empress 2, In-Ceram and Procera.

Biological Properties
They provide excellent marginal seal and exhibit a low incidence of post-operative sensitivity. The prolonged fluoride release provides anti-microbial and possibly anti-cariogenic properties, although clinical evidence for this property is lacking. These agents may contain the resin HEMA, which is a potent allergen - hence a no-touch technique should be used.

Limited research indicates that these agents should not be used in proximity to human pulpal tissue and should not be used where the pulp is within 1mm of the surface of the preparation.

Ease of Use
These materials are relatively user-friendly and associated with low incidence of post-operative sensitivity. Although moisture control is important, they are simpler to use and less technique-sensitive than resin cements. They should not be used with low-strength ceramics, but present information indicates that they may be utilised for high-strength materials, such as Procera, AllCeram, Inceram and Empress 2.

Provisional or Temporary Luting Agents

In addition to the ideal properties listed for 'permanent' luting cements, provisional cements have some further desired requirements. These include:

- Reduced mechanical properties, facilitating easy removal of restorations; yet it must not be so weak that it deforms or fractures during the provisional period.
- Allow minor tooth realignment within the provisional restoration.
- Do not interfere with polymerisation (for additions) or plasticise the provisional material.
- Do not discolour the provisional material.
- Do not alter the dental substrate (for instance, enamel, dentine or cementum).
- Do not adhere or adhere weakly to dental substrate and/or provisional materials.
- Provide therapeutic effects on traumatised pulps.
- Provide enhanced antimicrobial effects.

Zinc Oxide and Eugenol Cements
Tempbond®, Tempak®
These are traditional, non-reinforced cements that are cheap, easily mixed with non-specialised instruments (spatula and waxed pad or glass slab) and

form a thin cement thickness. They are markedly antimicrobial and exert an obtundent effect on pulp through the remaining dentinal thickness. They should not be used in contact with pulpal tissue (remaining dentinal thickness >1mm optimal). They provide ease of removal due to low tensile strength and lack of adhesion.

Eugenol leaching from the unset or set cement may cause discolouration of resin provisional materials and may inhibit polymerisation of additions. This is enhanced when the concentration of eugenol is increased. It is therefore recommended to use the manufacturer's proportions exactly (or even slightly reduce the eugenol proportion).

Eugenol absorbed into dentine and/or enamel may interfere with diffusion and polymerisation of adhesive resin-bonding systems and/or cements. Despite conflicting evidence on the clinical relevance of this effect, it is prudent to use alternative materials when the definitive restoration is to be adhesively luted.

These cements are strongly antimicrobial initially, but this property is lost over two to three weeks, as the eugenol leaches out. This makes it essential that all excess should be removed from the marginal area, especially subgingivally. Failure to remove subgingival excess will lead to plaque adhesion and subsequent inflammation. In delicate gingival tissues, this may lead to permanent changes (for instance, recession).

If provisional restorations are to be re-cemented all residual cement should be removed and the restoration thoroughly cleaned. This is readily accomplished by the use of a sandblaster and low pressure. This will remove all the material and roughen the resin surface, aiding in additions of fresh resin.

Non-Eugenol Cements
No-Genol®
This group of materials has similar physical and mechanical properties as their eugenol-containing relatives. They have reduced effects on resin polymerisation and discolouration. They have been shown, however, to interfere with adhesive agents and adhesive cements and therefore should be thoroughly cleaned from the tooth before bonding.

Polycarboxylate Cement
Ultratemp®
A weakened form of this hydrophilic cement is available for temporisation. It has the advantages of weak adhesion to tooth structure (sealing the denti-

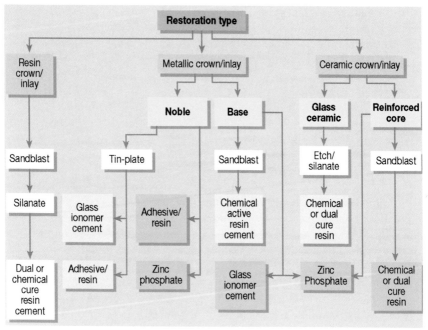

Fig 9-1 Luting options for indirect restorations.

nal surface), minimal effects on provisional resin materials and adhesive luting agents, and relative ease of removal. Thorough removal of all cement should be ensured before try-in of definitive restorations.

Conclusion

No available cement possesses ideal properties, as outlined (Fig 9-1). However, an understanding of the physical, mechanical and biological properties of individual cements permits their optimal use in differing clinical situations (Table 9-1).

Table 9-1 **Properties of luting cements**

	Mechanical	Physical	Adhesion	Antimicrobial/ Anti-cariogenic	Moisture Sensitivity	Application
ZnPO4	Moderate	Opaque. Powder/liquid	None	Nil after set	Moderate	All full-coverage restorations and metallic partial coverage restorations
GIC	Moderate to poor	Relatively opaque. Powder/liquid formulations	Tooth structure, tin-plated metal	Prolonged anti-cariogenic, possible anti-microbial	Moderate initial, needs barrier of resin or varnish	Similar to above (best avoided in high stress situations)
RMGI	Moderate	Increased translucency. Powder/liquid. Low solubility. Post-cure moisture absorption, causing expansion.	Tooth structure, tin-plated metal	Prolonged anti-cariogenic, possible anti-microbial properties	Moderate to low, advise barrier of resin or varnish but of less importance	Similar to above, avoid for conventional ceramic restorations
Resin	Good	Insoluble, best appearance. Paste/paste formulations	Highest bond strengths to etched/primed tooth, ceramic, base metal & primed noble alloy	Little or no anti-microbial or anti-cariogenic properties.	Very susceptible to moisture damage prior to set. Little effect post-setting.	All restorations where good moisture control can be achieved
Compomer	Moderate to good	Low solubility. Post-cure moisture absorption, causing expansion	Bonds to primed tooth structure	Initial anti-micro-bial effect but little after initial fluoride ion release	Reduced susceptibility compared with resins. Relative ease of use	Similar to resin cement but avoid with low strength ceramics
ZOE	Poor	Paste/paste opaque	No adhesion	Anti-microbial	High solubility	All materials except resin bonded
Poly-carboxylate	Moderate	Powder/liquid or paste/paste. Relative handling difficulty	Similar to GIC & RMGI	No anti-microbial effect	Moderate	Temporisation. Superseded by other materials for permanent lute

Further Reading

Hotz P, McLean JW, Sced I, Wilson AD. The bonding of glass ionomer cements to metal and tooth substrates. Br Dent J 1977;142:41-47.

Johnson GH, Powell LV, DeRouen TA. Evaluation and control of post-cementation pulpal sensitivity: zinc phosphate and glass ionomer luting cements. J Am Dent Assoc 1993;124:38-46.

Leinfelder KF. Current developments in dentin bonding systems: major progress found in today's products. J Am Dent Assoc 1993;124:40-42.

Pashley EL, Tao L, Matthews WG, Pashley DH. Bond strengths to superficial, intermediate and deep dentin in vivo with four dentine-bonding systems. Dent Mater 1993;9:19-22.

Peddey M. The bond strength of polycarboxylic acid cements to dentine: effect of surface modification and time after extraction. Aust Dent J 1981;26:178-180.

Piwowarczyk A, Lauer HC. Mechanical properties of luting cements after water storage. Oper Dent 2003;28:535-542.

Shimada Y, Yamaguchi S, Tagami J. Micro-shear bond strength of dual-cured resin cement to glass ceramic. Dental Material 2002;18:380-388.

Suzuki S. Clinical evaluation of a new resin composite crown system to eliminate postoperative sensitivity. Int J Periodontics Restorative Dent 2000;20:498-509.

Wilson AD, Batchelor RF. Zinc oxide-eugenol cements: II. Study of erosion and disintegration. J Dent Res. 1970;49:593-598.

Wilson AD, Kent BE, Lewis BG. Zinc phosphate cements: chemical study of in-vitro durability. J Dent Res 1970;49:1049-1054.

Wilson AD. Resin-modified glass-ionomer cements. Int J Prosthodont 1990;3:425-429.

Chapter10
Resin-Bonded Restorations

Aim

To review the factors involved in improving success rates of resin-bonded fixed partial dentures (RBFPD). The chapter will principally focus on tooth-related factors and RBFPD design. Resin cements are discussed in Chapter 9.

Outcome

This chapter underlines the fundamental tenet in RBFPD design that cement needs to be protected from tensile/shear forces in the same way as a conventional prosthesis, using principles of resistance and retention form in order to improve success.

Tooth-Related Factors

The most important tooth-related factors are:
- The amount of available enamel for bonding.
- Occlusal loading.

Amount of Available Enamel for Bonding
Any feature that increases the area for bonding, principally to enamel, will increase the retention of the prosthesis.
- *Tooth morphology* - the form of the palatal/lingual surface is the most significant feature. Teeth vary widely in terms of their mesio-distal and inciso-gingival dimensions. A maxillary lateral incisor offers less enamel surface than a maxillary central incisor, in the same way that the lingual aspect of a mandibular molar is poorer than the equivalent surface of a maxillary molar.
- *Tooth geometry* - the greater the area for bonding, the more force required to dislodge the RBFPD.
- *Available enamel* - any factor that reduces the amount of enamel available for bonding reduces the prognosis of the restoration (Fig 10-1). Enamel is lost primarily through caries, the presence of restorative material or by erosion and attrition. It has been found that the presence of restorations adversely affected clinical RBFPD success (Dunne and Millar 1993). In

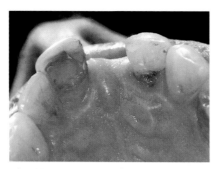

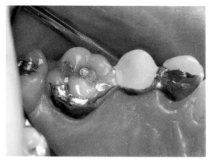

Fig 10-1 Amount of available enamel for bonding. The previous resin bonded prosthesis probably failed as a result of the limited enamel available on the central incisor due to the composite resin restoration. Note that the initial debond occurred on the central incisor clinically but that a partial debond on the lateral incisor resulted in dental caries.

Fig 10-2 Tooth-guided movements. This restoration repeatedly debonded on the canine tooth. This was probably caused by insufficient palatal coverage and the absence of grooves resulting in the mandibular canine forcing the maxillary canine facially during tooth-guided movement (note the wear facet). This resulted in shear stress that is poorly withstood by current luting agents.

the same way dentine exposure, with less predictable bonding, was found to reduce success. Thinning of the enamel layer and a decrease in the area of enamel available reduces the force required to dislodge the RBFPD. However, the presence of restorations may be used to increase the resistance and retention forms of the preparation – for instance, the incorporation of a proximal box into the framework as a result of removal of an existing Class 2 restoration.

- *Quality of enamel* - regional variation exists within enamel, with cervical enamel being least favourable. Crystal formation in this area is poorer, the resultant etch pattern is not as predictable, and bond strength reduced.

Occlusal Loading

- Occlusal contacts - occlusal contacts on RBFPDs should apply compressive rather than shearing forces. The compressive strength of a commonly used resin cement (Panavia F) is 200–300 MPa, whereas the tensile strength is only 20–40 MPa. High shear stresses are generated when:
  - A deep vertical overlap (overbite) exists on a retainer and a patient completes a lateral movement.
  - During a tooth-guided movement the contacting tooth moves from the metal retainer onto the tooth enamel. This may cause the abutment to be 'pushed away' from the retainer (Fig 10-2).

- Tooth contacts occur on the pontic during tooth-guided movements. This causes the pontic to be pushed facially and apically and exerts shear stress on the resin lute on the retainers.

• Presence of parafunction - occlusal factors that increase shear forces on resin cements retaining RBFPDs include forceful clenching and grinding of the teeth, in particular if deflective contacts are present in the pontic area. However, evidence for this is empirical, as no studies are available. Careful clinical and laboratory analysis of the static and dynamic occlusions and the adequacy of the maximum intercusping position (MIP), prior to tooth preparation, is required. This may highlight any prosthetic design alterations or modifications to the dentition that may result in more favourable loading on the RBFPD. In addition, the use of protective occlusal devices after placement of a RBFPD may decrease shear loading.

• Presence of oral habits - habits such as nail biting or the holding of pens, pins or nails between the teeth need to be identified and ceased before treatment. These habits generate high local stresses on the prosthesis.

Resin Luting Agents

Types
The most commonly employed resin cements are chemically cured or dual-cured bis-GMA or 4-META/MMA resins. These provide a stable bond and have been demonstrated to provide predictable success rates when used in clinical studies. Panavia EX (Kuraray, Japan) is the most commonly used bis-GMA cement, with reported laboratory-tested bond strengths to enamel in the region of 35-100 MPa and has been demonstrated to be significantly more successful in retaining RBFPDs than other cements.

C&B Metabond (Parkell, USA) is a 4-META/MMA resin that also has demonstrated high success rates over periods of up to 11 years, and develops bond strengths similar to Panavia. It has the advantage that it bonds to dentine with a hybrid layer and may be used to bond noble alloys to enamel or dentine.

Accuracy of Fit
The accuracy of fit of base metal alloys can be improved by applying the wax patterns directly to refractory dies instead of using the standard 'pulled' wax patterns and stone dies. This allows the wax-up of the RBFPD framework to be invested and cast directly on the refractory die. The adaptation of wax patterns to dies is superior to the adaptation of resin patterns to dies.

Cement Lute Thickness

A decrease in mean tensile strength with increasing cement thickness was observed *in vitro* for commonly used cements. Therefore the more accurate the adaptation of the prosthesis to the tooth, the greater the adhesive strength.

RBFPD Design and Tooth Preparation

Design of Metal Frameworks

Factors that contribute to resistance and retention include prosthesis rigidity, placement of grooves, parallelism of preparations, preparation design and finish.

Prosthesis Rigidity

Base metal alloys (nickel-chromium or cobalt-chromium) are optimal for RBFPDs because of their high modulus of elasticity and high tensile strengths. Their rigidity allows them to be very durable when used in thin sections for retainers and connectors. However, their low density and high melting point causes difficulty in casting the fine margins accurately, and they demonstrate inferior marginal fit compared to noble alloys. Their hardness makes it difficult to adjust and polish these alloys at the chairside. A strong predictable bond of base metal frameworks to resin cements can be achieved simply by sandblasting the fitting surface of the retainer. Increased thickness of retainer material prevents flexion of the framework and application of tensile forces to the cement bond.

Groove Placement

The addition of proximal grooves increased the force required to debond 0.5mm-thick retainers cemented with Panavia to metal dies of maxillary teeth. This involved an increase of 77% for lateral incisors, 31% for central incisors and 37% for canines. Clinical studies have confirmed this observation. Groove placement has furthermore been reported to improve the clinical success of posterior RBFPDs from 60% to 95% over a four-year period.

Parallelism of Preparations

When retainers with total convergence angles of 0 to 20 degrees were tested under laboratory conditions the more parallel retainers demonstrated a higher force to debond. Parallelism less than 5-10 degrees carries a risk of generating undercuts in the preparation. The generation of undercuts may lead to problems with seating the prosthesis and significant clinical time loss, as base metal is difficult to adjust.

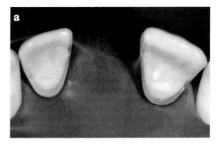

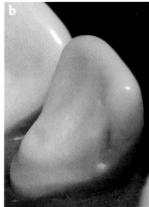

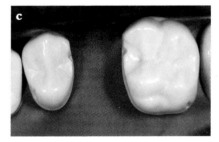

Fig 10-3 Suggested design and groove placement for RBFPDs. (a–b) Anterior and (c) posterior.

Preparation Design
Posterior Design (Fig 10-3 and Fig 10-4)
Key features identified as critical for fixed partial denture survival are:

- The surface area covered by the metal and the design were significant in affecting bond strength and durability.
- Occlusal coverage improved resistance and retention.
- Grooves increased the force required to cause failure. Whether this was due to increased bond strength (increased area of enamel), increased retention form or increased rigidity of the casting or a combination of these factors is unclear. The ideal retainer design should have lingual wrap-around (>180 degrees), occlusal coverage and grooves sited diametrically opposite each other. Occlusal coverage is convenient on mandibular first premolars, where the lingual cusp is relatively small, but more difficult on other mandibular or maxillary teeth.

Anterior Design (Fig 10-3 and Fig 10-4)
Two schools of thought exist as to the incisal extent of metal coverage on anterior teeth. The first is that the metal should stop up to 2mm short of the incisal edge to avoid loss of abutment translucency. This is more critical in incisors than canine teeth. The disadvantage of this approach is that, if tooth-guided movement along the retainer moves forcefully from the metal to

133

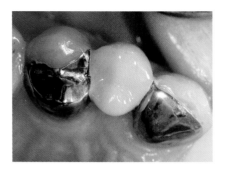

Fig 10-4 Suggested retainer design. Retainers should cover the maximum area including the occlusal surface where possible. Retainers should be 0.5mm thick as standard, as shown on this restoration immediately post-luting, prior to final finishing.

tooth, high shear stresses may result. These stresses may be better resisted, in theory, using proximal grooves. The second approach is to extend the metal to the incisal edge, ensuring that tooth-guided movements are only on the retainer, limiting shear stresses on the cement. The extent of 'greying out' of the incisal edge can be assessed before preparation using a white paste on a metal matrix band. The base portion of setting calcium hydroxide preparations is a readily available paste for this purpose.

Number of Abutments and Pontics
The presence of more than two abutments or more than one pontic increases the clinical rate of failure of RBFPDs (Fig 10-5). This may be related to the law of beam, according to which, increased flexibility of longer-span pontic frameworks is to be expected for frameworks of the same cross-sectional width.

Cantilever Resin-Bonded FPDs

Cantilever design evolved from the observation of partial failure of RBFPDs with two abutment teeth, where one retainer, usually the smaller, debonded. The debonded retainer was removed and the RBFPD left *in situ*. Anecdotally, a large proportion of these prostheses functioned well, creating interest in cantilever prostheses. The advantage of cantilever RBFPDs is that it removes the differential bond strength due to the differing size and mobility of the abutments (Fig 10-6).

Debonding of cantilever RBFPDs is immediately obvious to the patient, as the prosthesis is dislodged. If two retainers exist on a prosthesis and one debonds, the patient may not be aware of the failure. Rapid caries progression in these instances has been reported.

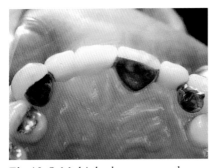

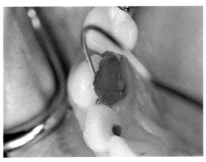

Fig 10-5 Multiple abutments and pontics. Greater than two abutments or more than one pontic increase the clinical rate of failure of RBFPDs. This restoration has a poor prognosis for these reasons, in addition to the poor retainer design.

Fig 10-6 Failure of RBFPDs. Cantilever design evolved from the failure of such three unit restorations.

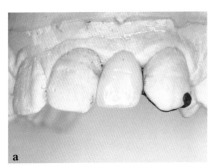

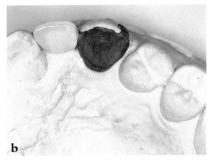

Fig 10-7 (a-b) Cantilever RBFPD retainer design. The retainer should cover maximum area, be of 0.5mm thickness and have greater than 180° 'wrap-around'. An incisal hook facilitates correct seating of the restoration at the luting stage.

The disadvantages of cantilever RBFPDs are that they are more difficult to cement accurately in position and may require additional features such as incisal hooks for positioning (Fig 10-7). They may not be suitable for post-orthodontic patients or those who have extensive loss of periodontal attachment where the potential for unplanned tooth movement exists (Figs 10-8). Furthermore, if the prosthesis debonds there is a risk of ingestion /inhalation.

Clinical studies of cantilever designs have demonstrated a debond rate as low as 6% over 36 months. The most frequently reported cantilever RBFPD

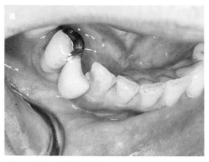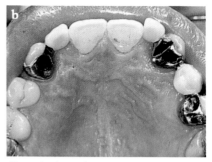

Fig 10-8 CRBFPD restorations are not indicated where there is a potential for (a) tooth drift due to attachment loss or (b) relapse of previous orthodontic tooth movement.

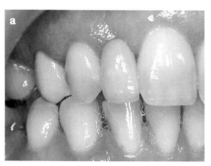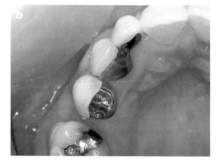

Fig 10-9 (a-b) Cantilever RBFPDs provide predictable restorations, in particular when replacing maxillary lateral incisors. Note that the 'wrap-around' on the canine tooth is greater than 180° as the restoration on the premolar was being placed at the same time.

type was the replacement of a maxillary lateral incisor, using a canine as the abutment (Fig 10-9).

Conclusions

In conclusion the following factors may enhance success rates of RBFPDs:
- Careful case selection: looking at factors such as available enamel, tooth form, occlusal loading, and area of periodontal attachment of the abutment(s).
- Use of refractory dies to fabricate metal castings.
- Coverage of the maximum area of enamel.
- Coverage of a portion of the occlusal surface if feasible.

- Increased retainer thickness, ≥0.5mm.
- Placement of parallel grooves.
- Creation of near–parallel preparations.
- Single tooth replacement only.
- Avoidance of double abutments or two abutments of differing size/stability.
- Cantilever RBFPDs offer comparable success rates to standard RBFPDs and should be considered for the replacement of maxillary lateral incisors and areas where differential mobility of abutments exist.

Further Reading

Barrack G, Bretz WA. A long–term prospective study of the etched–cast restoration. Int J Prosthodont 1993;6:428-434.

Djemal S, Setchell D, King P, Wickens J. Long–term survival characteristics of 832 resin–retained bridges and splints provided in a post–graduate teaching hospital between 1978 and 1993. J Oral Rehabil 1999;26:302-320.

Dunne SM, Millar BJ. A longitudinal study of the clinical performance of resin bonded bridges and splints. Br Dent J 1993;174:405-411.

El Salam Shakal MA, Pfeiffer P, Hilgers RD. Effect of tooth preparation design on bond strengths of resin–bonded prostheses: a pilot study. J Prosthet Dent 1997;77:243-249.

Hussey DL, Linden GJ. The clinical performance of cantilevered resin–bonded bridgework. J Dent 1996;24:251-256.

Chapter 11
Restoration of Non-Vital Teeth

Aim

This chapter presents a strategy for assessing non-vital teeth for restoration and the range of restorative options available to practitioners. The relative merits of each approach are outlined.

Outcome

At the end of this chapter the practitioner should understand that endodontically treated teeth are weakened because part of the tooth structure is removed during preparation and instrumentation. The main reasons why teeth lose vitality, such as caries and trauma, frequently result in the loss of tooth structure. In addition, non-vital teeth may be somewhat more brittle than vital teeth. Because non-vital teeth are compromised, the main objectives when restoring are to maintain the tooth integrity and function and to achieve an aesthetic result. In order to preserve the tooth, every effort is made to leave the apical seal intact and to prevent subsequent fracture of the tooth.

Diagnostic Considerations for the Restoration of Non-Vital Teeth

The same general considerations apply to the restoration of non-vital teeth as to vital teeth, such as the general and oral health of the patient, cost and time involved (see Chapter 1). There are some issues that are particularly important for, and specific to, the successful restoration of non-vital teeth:

- *Successful endodontic treatment* – absence of clinical signs of periapical infection. No tenderness to percussion. No swelling, tenderness or exudate around the root of the tooth. Radiographic evidence of intact, or healing, periapical bone.
- *Tooth is restorable* – no evidence of root fracture. Sufficient tooth structure remaining to provide a predictable restoration.
- *Good periodontal status* – bone levels around the tooth sufficient to support a post, where needed.
- *Favourable occlusion* – teeth that are subject to parafunction or repeated occlusal trauma may have a poorer prognosis.

- *Protection from trauma* – teeth that have been traumatised, or are at risk of repeated trauma, such as in contact sports, will have an increased chance of restoration failure or root fracture.
- *Independent of other restorations* – fixed and removable partial dentures may have a poorer prognosis when the abutment teeth are endodontically treated.

Selection of the Restoration for a Non-Vital Tooth

Not every non-vital tooth requires extensive restoration and, in general, the simpler the restoration provided, the better (Table 11-1). Initial questions include:
- Does the tooth require a crown?
- Does the tooth require a post and core?
- If so, what type of post and core?

The decision to restore a non-vital tooth, or which type of restoration is appropriate, depends mainly on:
- Location of tooth in the arch.
- Amount of tooth structure remaining.
- Root size and morphology.
- Use of the tooth as an abutment.

Anterior Teeth

Endodontically Treated Anterior Teeth
Does the Tooth Need a Crown?
Endodontically treated anterior teeth are structurally weakened due to the access cavity and instrumentation of the root canal. They often have associated tooth loss caused by fractures, caries or existing restorations. There is little evidence to suggest that providing a crown on anterior teeth by itself increases the clinical survival of the tooth. Therefore, the coronal part of the tooth may be restored with a composite resin restoration, provided there is sufficient tooth structure remaining to retain the restoration, sufficient dentine to resist coronal fracture, and the shade of the remaining tooth is acceptable (Fig 11-1).

Sealing the Root Canal
When an endodontically treated tooth is restored with a composite resin restoration, it is important that leakage through the coronal part of the root canal be prevented. This may be accomplished by removing 2-3mm of root filling apical to the cementoenamel junction and placing a seal, such as a glass

Table 11-1 **A guide for definitive restoration of endodontically treated teeth**

Status of coronal structure (Following removal of caries and existing restorations)	Suggested restoration
Access cavity only	Composite resin restoration
At least two thirds of crown remaining	Composite resin restoration
Mild to moderate discolouration and at least two thirds of crown remaining	Bleaching or labial veneer plus composite resin restoration
Less than two thirds of crown remaining	Full crown
Severe discolouration	Full crown

Fig 11-1
(a) Destruction of coronal tissue, which could be restored with a composite resin restoration. (b) Loss of coronal tissue, which requires restoration with a crown.

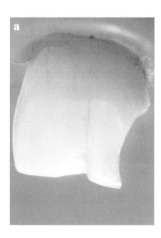 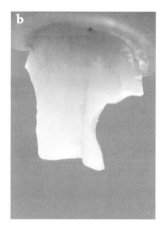

ionomer restoration, in the root canal (Fig 11-2). This will ensure that bacteria from the oral environment (for example, from leakage of a composite filling) will not penetrate the root.

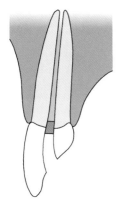

Fig 11-2 Sealing the root canal of an endodontically treated tooth with a glass ionomer material.

Internal Bleaching
Internal bleaching of a discoloured endodontically treated tooth may be indicated where at least two thirds of the tooth crown remains and the discolouration is not severe. When the adjacent teeth have a high degree of translucency or colouration, then bleaching may not match these teeth successfully, since it tends to produce a whitish crown, which is relatively opaque. If the tooth is to be bleached internally, it is essential that the root canal be properly sealed against the bleaching chemicals, which may cause cervical root resorption (see above).

A protocol for internal bleaching is as follows:
- Remove caries and discoloured fillings. Clear access cavity and seal the root canal.
- Make a bleaching paste from water and sodium perborate powder (Bocasan, Oral B).
- Fill the access cavity with bleaching paste and seal the cavity with glass ionomer cement.
- Review the discolouration after a week. The bleaching paste may be replaced a second or third time.
- If a satisfactory shade is achieved, then remove the bleaching paste and restore the tooth with a composite resin restoration.
- For darker teeth it may be advisable to over-bleach the tooth to allow for some regression of the shade.

Does the Tooth Need a Post and Core?
If a crown is required for successful restoration of the tooth, then the next

142

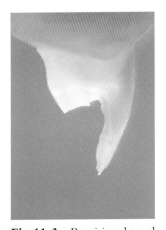

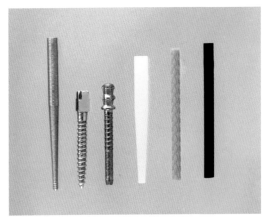

Fig 11-3 Provisional tooth preparation shows insufficient structure remains to retain a crown.

Fig 11-4 Selection of endodontic posts. (From left) tapered titanium post (Filhol), tapered threaded post (Dentatus), serrated/threaded parallel post (Parapost XT), glass– fibre post (Postec), serrated plastic parallel impression post (Parapost), smooth plastic parallel impression post (Parapost).

decision is whether or not a post and core is required. A core will be required if there is insufficient tooth structure remaining to retain a crown or if the dentine is so weakened that a coronal fracture is likely to occur. This is a somewhat subjective decision, and it will depend on the amount and location of the remaining tooth structure and the type of crown to be placed. The balance of evidence suggests that a post itself does not reinforce the remaining tooth; the main role for the post is to provide retention for the core material. It is helpful to first prepare the tooth for the crown and then evaluate the amount of dentine remaining (Fig 11-3). If, after crown preparation, there is sufficient bulk of well-supported dentine to retain a crown a post and core may not be required.

What Type of Post and Core should I Use?
A wide variety of post and core systems has been developed in almost every combination of material, shape and surface (Fig 11-4). This suggests that none has a clear advantage, although some consideration should be given to match the post type to the clinical situation (Table 11-2). The root size and morphology and the type of final restoration planned for the tooth will influence this decision.

In order to place a metal-ceramic crown on a maxillary central incisor with

Table 11-2 **Properties of various posts and cores types**

Post and core type	Features
Cast post and core	The most versatile, as it can be made to fit tapered, irregular or angulated root canals. Cast core can replace extensive loss of coronal dentine.
Prefabricated post with core build-up	May save time and can be completed in a single visit. Relatively inexpensive. Does not fit all canal types

Post and core material	Features
Cast metal	Accurate fit of canal. Usually noble alloy. Non-precious alloys may corrode.
Prefabricated metal	Rigid and strong. Usually stainless steel or titanium. Does not bond well to composite.
Carbon fibre	Modulus of elasticity similar to dentine. Retrievable. May bond to dentine. Dark colour may show through root.
Glass/quartz fibre	No discolouration of tooth. Less rigid than carbon fibre. Retrievable. May bond to dentine.
Ceramic	Zirconium with composite or pressed ceramic core. Aesthetic and very rigid. Difficult to retrieve if fractured.

Post shape	Features
Parallel	Retentive. Requires preparation of root canal.
Tapered	Less retentive than parallel post. May need less removal of tooth structure in apical third.

Post surface	Features
Serrated	More retentive than smooth-sided.
Smooth	Adequate in most situations.
Threaded	Most retentive post but increases risk of root fracture.

a wide tapering root canal and extensive coronal destruction, a cast-metal post and core would probably be a good choice. For a maxillary lateral incisor with good coronal structure, which is to be restored with an all-ceramic crown, a prefabricated glass fibre post with a composite core could be used successfully.

Tooth Preparation for Post and Core
The main principle in preparing a tooth for a post and core is to maintain as much tooth structure as possible while removing any thin or undermined areas of dentine, which are likely to fracture (Fig 11-5). Several studies suggest that the presence of 2-3mm of sound dentine coronal to the crown finish line is the key factor in strengthening the final crown-post-tooth assembly. The greater the coronal structure remaining on the tooth, the less significant is the type of post and core used to provide additional retention. The preservation of coronal dentine also ensures that the core-tooth junction is incisal to the crown-tooth junction, which helps prevent leakage from the oral environment into the root canal.

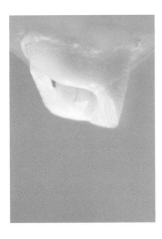

Fig 11-5 Coronal preparation of central incisor for a post and core.

Principles of tooth preparation of coronal tooth structure are to:
- Carefully remove any caries or unsound restorations.
- Prepare the crown finish line. The details of the finish line depend on the type of crown that will be placed on the tooth.
- Remove walls of dentine that are less than 1mm thick or are undermined.
- Remove unevenness from the incisal surface of the preparation so the core will have a definite surface to finish on.
- Proceed with preparation of the root canal for a post.

The main objectives in preparing the root canal space for a post are to preserve the apical seal in the root canal and to minimise the removal of tooth structure while allowing sufficient strength for the post restoration. In order to avoid perforation of the root during preparation, it is important to first be familiar with the size and angulation of the root using clinical observation and radiographs.

The longer a post, the more retentive it will be and the less stress concentration will occur in the root. In general, posts should extend into the root of a tooth as far as possible without disturbing the apical root canal filling. Studies indicate that at least 4mm of apical gutta percha filling should remain in the root canal to ensure an adequate apical seal. Assuming that the root filling extends close to the root apex, a post length equal to the root length minus 4mm will be sufficient in almost all cases (Table 11-3). The preservation of coronal tooth structure also adds to the effective length of the post.

Table 11-3 **Standard root length for anterior teeth**

| | Average root length (CEJ to Apex) | | |
	Central incisor	Lateral incisor	Canine
Maxilla	13	13	17
Mandible	12.5	14	15

Principles of canal preparation are:
- Preparation of the post space should be completed with rubber dam in place.
- Information recorded from the endodontic treatment and from radiographs of the tooth should be used to establish the post length.
- The root-canal filling should be removed from the post space using safe-ended drills, such as Peeso reamers or Gates-Glidden drills (Fig 11-6).
- A rubber stopper should be used to mark the length of post space on the drill.
- The drill should be used only at slow speed when removing the root-canal filling.
- A drill size that will easily fit within the root canal should be used initially.
- Gentle force should be applied to the drill in an apical direction to avoid perforation of the root canal.
- If the drill meets resistance in the root canal, stop and reassess the angulation of the drill (Fig 11-7).
- Increasing diameters of drills should be used to remove the remainder of the root canal filling.

Fig 11-6 Parapost twist drill (top) for parallel preparation of the root canal. Peeso reamer (centre) and Gates-Glidden drill (bottom) for removal of gutta percha endodontic filling material. Note the use of silicone stoppers and a millimetre ruler to measure the length of root-canal preparation.

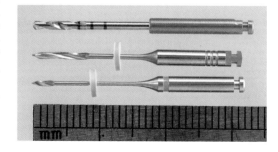

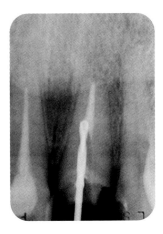

Fig 11-7 Assessment of root-canal preparation. Deviation of the twist drill from the root canal with a risk of root perforation.

After removal of the root-canal filling the post space can be completed. Twist drills are supplied with the post system being used and come in a range of diameters. The drills are used to achieve the final shape and diameter preparation for the post (Fig 11-6). As a general rule, the diameter of the preparation should not leave less than 1mm of dentine surrounding the post. This is to protect against root fracture and root perforation. However, it is not usually necessary to achieve the greatest possible post diameter, especially where there is coronal tooth structure remaining.

As a guide:
- In most anterior teeth, a post with a diameter of 1.25mm or less is sufficiently strong, and a wider diameter post is not significantly more retentive.
- When the root canal itself is wider than 1.25mm a wider post will be required, although the canal preparation should be limited to the removal of undercuts.
- Frequently a root canal tapers apically, in which case only the apical third to half needs to be prepared with the twist drill, and the coronal part of the canal should be cleaned and smoothed.
- If the post and core preparation provides no resistance to rotation an anti-rotational groove should be placed in the coronal third of the tooth preparation.

Impression for a Post and Core

Either a direct or indirect impression may be made for the post and core. The direct impression involves making a pattern for the final post and core directly on the tooth with resin or wax. The advantage of the direct impression is that the clinician has control over the size and shape of the post and core - for example, to make sure that the entire post space is utilised and the core is correctly orientated. The disadvantage of the direct technique is that it is relatively time-consuming clinically, and if any difficulty arises with the post and core pattern in the laboratory a new impression must be made. The indirect approach uses an elastic impression material to take an impression of the tooth preparation, which is then sent to the laboratory, where a post and core pattern is made.

Direct Technique (Fig 11-8)
- The post space is lightly lubricated.
- Plastic impression posts are usually supplied with the post kit to match the sizes of the twist drills.
- A post is selected that is the same diameter as the largest twist drill used for the post space preparation.
- Serrated impression posts may be used to improve the retention of the post and core.
- The impression post is tried in the canal and resin is added to the coronal part of the post as it is seated.
- Resin is added incrementally to the pattern to create a snug fit with the post space.
- Ensure removal of the post pattern several times while the resin is setting, so the pattern does not get stuck in the root canal.
- Once the post pattern has achieved initial set, begin adding resin to form the core.
- When completely set, the core may be shaped with high-speed diamond burs under copious water spray.
- Resistance of the post and core pattern to rotation may be easily assessed at this stage. If necessary, the anti-rotational features of the preparation can be increased.
- The completed post and core pattern is removed and sent to the laboratory for casting.

Indirect Technique
- The post space is lightly lubricated.
- A smooth-sided plastic impression post is selected that is just smaller than the post space.
- Allow the impression post to protrude 5-7mm from the tooth when fully seated.
- Bend or serrate the top of the impression post, or add a ball of resin, so that the post will be firmly retained in the impression.

149

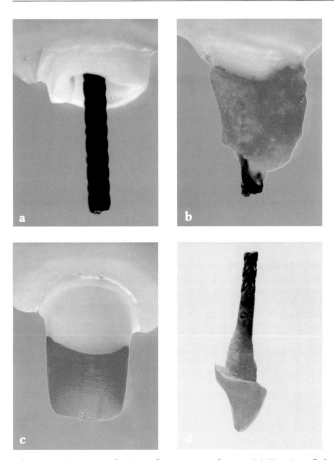

Fig 11-8 Direct technique for a post and core. (a) Try-in of plastic impression post to match the twist drill used for root canal preparation. (b) Pattern resin applied to the impression post to build up the core structure. (c) The post and core pattern is trimmed to the required shape. (d) Completed pattern is removed and sent to the laboratory to be cast.

- Coat the impression post with adhesive for the impression material.
- Syringe silicone impression material into the post space and use an endodontic spiral filler to fill the space completely.
- Insert the impression post into the canal and seat it fully.
- Place the loaded impression tray over the teeth.
- When the impression is fully set, remove the impression carefully, complete with post.

- The impression is sent to the laboratory with instructions for fabrication of the post and core.

Posts should be made from a material that is rigid, tough and resistant to corrosion. Most posts and cores are made from cast metal - commonly gold alloys or silver-palladium alloys. Alloys with a high modulus of elasticity should be selected, but base-metal alloys should be avoided because of their corrosion potential. If the tooth is to be restored with a metal-ceramic crown the colour of the post and core may not be an important issue. If a ceramic crown is to be used a post system should be selected that will not detract from the final colouration of the crown. In this case, a gold-coloured alloy is more suitable than a silver or grey alloy. Alternatively, the labial surface of the metal core can be bonded with opaque porcelain to enhance its appearance.

A recent innovation is the all-ceramic post and core system. A prefabricated zirconium post is selected to match the prepared post space. Resin is added to the post to fill in the post space and to make up the core. The pattern is sent to the laboratory where the resin is replaced with a pressed ceramic material, resulting in a highly aesthetic post and core.

Cementation of Endodontic Posts

Traditionally, posts were cemented with luting agents, such as zinc phosphate, which do not provide a chemical bond between the post and the tooth. The luting of posts is clinically successful where the size and shape of the post is within the normal guidelines discussed above. The further advantage of luting agents is that they generally make it possible to remove the post, should it become necessary to provide endodontic treatment, or to replace the post. A common alternative to luting agents is to use a glass ionomer or polycarboxylate cement, which bonds chemically to metal posts and to dentine. However, the bond strength of the glass ionomers to dentine is relatively weak, so that the overall resistance of posts to removal is approximately the same as with the luting agents.

Resin cements are increasingly popular for the cementation of endodontic posts. These cements are strong and, when used with dentine bonding agents, can provide a bond between the post and the root. A bonded post may be a good option when extra retention of the post is desired - for example, in teeth with short roots or tapered root canals. It has been suggested that the bonding of a post to the tooth creates a 'bonded unit' that has increased resistance to fracture. However, there are no long-term clinical studies to clearly support the use of any cement or bonding system for endodontic posts.

Direct Post and Core

Anterior teeth that have at least 2-3mm of dentine incisal to the crown finish line may be restored directly with a prefabricated post and a composite resin core. The principles of the coronal and root preparations are the same as outlined for custom post and core systems.

Non-metallic posts have gained popularity recently for the direct restoration of endodontically treated teeth. Carbon, glass or quartz fibres are embedded in a resin matrix, and this composite material is formed into prefabricated posts. *In vitro* data suggest that the main advantage of the fibre post is that under high loads the post will fracture before the tooth, resulting in a 'safer' restoration. Carbon-fibre posts are dark in colour, and so may not be desirable aesthetically. Glass and quartz fibre posts are light in colour, so they will not discolour the final crown or be visible through the tooth structure.

All-ceramic posts, such as zirconium and alumina, have also been suggested as direct restorations. These materials are very rigid and are light in colour. Unlike the fibre-reinforced posts, the ceramic posts are extremely hard and so are difficult to cut intraorally. Fractured ceramic posts may be very difficult to remove when bonded to the tooth.

The usual approach to direct post and cores (Fig 11-9) is that:
• A post is selected to match the size of twist drill used for the post space preparation.
• Prefabricated posts are generally designed as bonded restorations. The exact procedures for bonding metal, fibre-reinforced, or ceramic posts should be followed according to the manufacturer's instructions.
• The core is built up on the bonded post and trimmed.
• The post is cut to the full length of the post and core restoration.
• After final shaping of the core, an impression is made for a crown on the tooth.

Posterior Teeth

Posterior teeth that have extensive loss of coronal tissue or finish lines extending subgingivally may be difficult to restore adequately. Endodontically treated posterior teeth are more susceptible to fracture than anterior teeth,

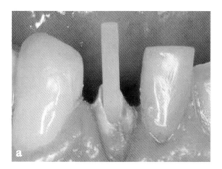
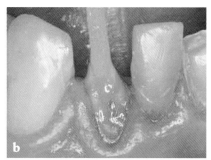
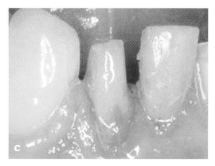

Fig 11-9 Direct placement of a non-metal post and core. (a) A glass-fibre post is selected to match the twist drill used for preparation of the post space. (b) Post is bonded to the tooth with bonding agent and resin cement. (c) Core build-up is completed with composite resin.

and some studies suggest that non-vital posterior teeth should routinely have cuspal coverage to prevent extensive fractures. As a general rule, it should be possible to place a crown finish line on sound dentine, with at least 2mm of dentine coronal to the finish line. This will provide good resistance for the coronal restoration, reducing its dependence on the endodontic posts and decreasing the likelihood of leakage from the oral cavity into the roots themselves (Table 11-4). If a restoration cannot be placed on sound tooth structure the long-term viability of the tooth must be questioned.

Axial Walls Mainly Intact

Where most of the tooth destruction has been within the crown, and three or four cusps are remaining (two cusps in the case of premolars) it is generally possible to restore the missing tooth structure with an amalgam or composite resin restoration (Fig 11-10).

Technique
- Remove caries and existing restorations from the crown of the tooth and the endodontic access cavity.

Table 11-4 **Guidelines for restoration of non-vital posterior teeth**

Status of coronal structure (Following removal of caries and existing restorations)	Suggested restoration
Axial walls mainly intact	Intracoronal amalgam or composite resin restoration. Cuspal coverage with partial or full crown.
Moderate loss of structure: at least half of axial walls intact	Amalgam or composite resin restoration with additional retention from endodontic post(s) with crown.
Severe loss of structure: less than half of axial walls intact	Cast post and core with crown.

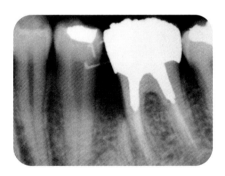

Fig 11-10 Amalgam core extending into the root canals for retention.

- Trim any thin (<2mm) or unsupported tooth structure.
- Check there is sufficient retention and resistance for the restoration provided by the remaining tooth.
- If necessary, use a small round bur to remove 2mm of gutta percha from the coronal part of each root canal.
- Condense the amalgam well into the root canal openings and proceed with incremental filling of the tooth.
- When set hard, or at the next visit, prepare the tooth for a full crown.

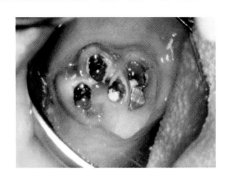

Fig 11-11 Three titanium posts cemented into the roots of a maxillary second molar for retention of an amalgam core.

Moderate Loss of Coronal Structure

Where half of the axial walls are intact - approximately two cusps in molars or one cusp in premolars - then the core build up in the tooth needs additional retention. This is to prevent the core from being dislodged during function and minimise leakage that could occur due to movement of the core. The core material may be amalgam or composite resin; each has particular advantages and disadvantages. Amalgam is strong, dimensionally stable and moisture-tolerant but may be unacceptable to some patients. Composite resin is very strong and may be bonded to the remaining dentine and to some endodontic posts. It has the advantage of rapid or command set, so it can be prepared for a crown at the same visit when at its placement. However, composite resin is often not dimensionally stable, and a large bulk of core material will shrink significantly on polymerisation, making the restoration liable to leakage. If exposed to the oral environment composite resin may absorb water, leading to expansion of the material and difficulty fitting the definitive crown.

Post-retained restorations in posterior teeth usually take advantage of the divergent roots to help retain the core material. As a general rule, it is desirable to place one post for each missing cusp of the tooth (Fig 11-11). Posts placed in one or more roots, together with the remaining coronal walls, provide good retention for the core and for the other posts. For this reason it is not usually necessary to make the posts as long as possible.

Technique
- Remove caries and existing restorations from the crown of the tooth and trim any thin (<2mm) or unsupported tooth structure.
- Using radiographs and endodontic records to check the root morphology, remove 5-6mm of gutta percha from each root canal that is to receive a post. Make sure there is at least 4-5mm of apical filling left in the canal.

- Use a twist drill to minimally prepare the post space so that a prefabricated post can be fitted.
- Trim a prefabricated post - metal or carbon/glass fibre - so that it extends from the root canal to within 1mm of the occlusal surface of the tooth.
- Cement the post in the root canal using a luting agent (for metal posts) or dentine bonding system (carbon or glass fibre).
- With a matrix band in place, build up the remainder of the core.
- When completely set, the tooth may be prepared for a full coverage restoration.
- The crown finish line should extend at least 2mm on sound tooth structure all around the tooth.

Severe Loss of Coronal Structure

When almost all the coronal dentine of a posterior tooth has been destroyed the final crown will depend on endodontic posts for retention. For this reason, maximum strength and rigidity of the post and core is needed. Prefabricated posts with a core build-up may be used, but the cores may not be sufficiently strong in thin sections surrounding the posts. An alternative is to use a cast post and core system but taking advantage of divergent roots, particularly in molars, to 'lock in' the restoration. Because of the complexity of these post and cores they are normally fabricated using an indirect technique (Fig 11-12).

Technique
- Prepare the remaining coronal tissue and access cavity in the same way as the moderate loss of structure (above).
- The larger canal in premolars and molars can be used for the main post and is prepared as for an anterior tooth.
- A small-size twist drill may be used to prepare the coronal part of the second or third root canals for accessory retention and resistance.

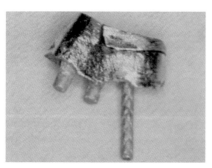

Fig 11-12 Two-piece cast post and core for a maxillary second molar with extensive coronal destruction.

156

- A size-matched impression pin is placed in each of the canals and an impression is made with an elastomeric material.
- In the laboratory, a two- or three-piece post and core casting is made. Frequently the main part of the core and the two smaller posts (buccal canals in maxillary molars or mesial canals in mandibular molars) form one casting, while the larger post slides through the main core to lock the whole assembly together on the tooth.
- The post and core casting is checked and cemented in place.
- The crown preparation on the tooth may be completed, but the finish line should extend 2mm onto sound tooth structure.

Conclusion

A wide variety of options exists for the restoration of endodontically treated teeth. Conservation of tooth structure, protection of the remaining tooth and prevention of leakage are important factors in the longevity of restorations. Most restorative materials will yield good results in non-vital teeth, provided that these basic principles are observed.

Further Reading

Fredriksson M, Astback J, Pamenius M, Arvidson K. A retrospective study of 236 patients with teeth restored by carbon fiber-reinforced epoxy resin posts. J Prosthet Dent 1998;80:151-157.

Goodacre CJ, Spolnik KJ. The prosthodontic management of endodontically treated teeth: a literature review. Part III. Tooth preparation considerations. J Prosthodont 1995;4:122-128.

Goodacre CJ, Spolnik KJ. The prosthodontic management of endodontically treated teeth: a literature review. Part II. Maintaining the apical seal. J Prosthodont 1995;4:51-53.

Goodacre CJ, Spolnik KJ. The prosthodontic management of endodontically treated teeth: a literature review. Part I. Success and failure data, treatment concepts. J Prosthodont 1994;3:243-250.

Isidor F, Brondum K, Ravnholt G. The influence of post length and crown ferrule length on the resistance to cyclic loading of bovine teeth with prefabricated titanium posts. Int J Prosthodont 1999;12:78-82.

Nayyar A, Walton RE, Leonard LA. An amalgam coronal-radicular dowel and core technique for endodontically treated posterior teeth. J Prosthet Dent 1980;43:511-515.

Sorensen JA, Martinoff JT. Clinically significant factors in dowel design. J Prosthet Dent 1984;52:28–35.

Sorensen JA, Martinoff JT. Endodontically treated teeth as abutments. J Prosthet Dent 1985;53:631–636.

Index

Quintessentials for General Dental Practitioners Series

in 36 volumes

Editor-in-Chief: Professor Nairn H F Wilson

The Quintessentials for General Dental Practitioners Series covers basic principles and key issues in all aspects of modern dental medicine. Each book can be read as a stand-alone volume or in conjunction with other books in the series.

Publication date, approximately

Oral Surgery and Oral Medicine, Editor: John G Meechan

Practical Dental Local Anaesthesia	available
Practical Oral Medicine	available
Practical Conscious Sedation	available
Practical Surgical Dentistry	Autumn 2005

Imaging, Editor: Keith Horner

Interpreting Dental Radiographs	available
Panoramic Radiology	Autumn 2005
Twenty-first Century Dental Imaging	Spring 2006

Periodontology, Editor: Iain L C Chapple

Understanding Periodontal Diseases: Assessment and Diagnostic Procedures in Practice	available
Decision-Making for the Periodontal Team	available
Successful Periodontal Therapy – A Non-Surgical Approach	available
Periodontal Management of Children, Adolescents and Young Adults	available
Periodontal Medicine: A Window on the Body	Autumn 2005

Implantology, Editor: Lloyd J Searson

Implantology in General Dental Practice	available
Managing Orofacial Pain in Practice	Spring 2006

Endodontics, Editor: John M Whitworth

Rational Root Canal Treatment in Practice	available
Managing Endodontic Failure in Practice	available
Managing Dental Trauma in Practice	Autumn 2005
Preventing Pulpal Injury in Practice	Autumn 2005

Prosthodontics, Editor: P Finbarr Allen

Teeth for Life for Older Adults	available
Complete Dentures – from Planning to Problem Solving	available
Removable Partial Dentures	available
Fixed Prosthodontics in Dental Practice	available
Occlusion: A Theoretical and Team Approach	Spring 2006

Operative Dentistry, Editor: Paul A Brunton

Decision-Making in Operative Dentistry	available
Aesthetic Dentistry	available
Indirect Restorations	Spring 2006
Communicating in Dental Practice: Stress Free Dentistry and Improved Patient Care	Spring 2006
Applied Dental Materials in Operative Dentistry	Spring 2006

Paediatric Dentistry/Orthodontics, Editor: Marie Therese Hosey

Child Taming: How to Cope with Children in Dental Practice	available
Paediatric Cariology	available
Treatment Planning for the Developing Dentition	Autumn 2005

General Dentistry and Practice Management, Editor: Raj Rattan

The Business of Dentistry	available
Risk Management	available
Practice Management for the Dental Team	Autumn 2005
Quality Matters: From Clinical Care to Customer Service	Autumn 2005
Dental Practice Design	Spring 2006
IT in Dentistry: A Working Manual	Spring 2006

Quintessence Publishing Co. Ltd., London